GYNAECOLOGY
by Ten Teachers

GYNAECOLOGY

by Ten Teachers

19th Edition

Edited By

Ash Monga BMED (SCI) BM BS MRCOG

Consultant Gynaecologist, Princess Anne Hospital,
Southampton University Hospitals NHS Trust,
Southampton, UK

Stephen Dobbs MD FRCOG

Consultant Gynaecological Oncologist,
Belfast City Hospital, Belfast Trust,
Belfast, UK

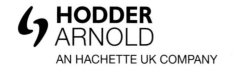

**HODDER
ARNOLD**
AN HACHETTE UK COMPANY

First published in Great Britain in 1919 as Diseases of Women
Eleventh edition published in 1966 as Gynaecology
Eighteenth edition published in 2006
This nineteenth edition published in 2011 by
Hodder Arnold, an imprint of Hodder Education, a division of Hachette UK,
338 Euston Road, London NW1 3BH

http://www.hodderarnold.com

© 2011 Hodder & Stoughton Ltd

Whilst the advice and information in this book are believed to be true and accurate at the date of going to press, neither the author[s] nor the publisher can accept any legal responsibility or liability for any errors or omissions that may be made. In particular (but without limiting the generality of the preceding disclaimer) every effort has been made to check drug dosages; however it is still possible that errors have been missed. Furthermore, dosage schedules are constantly being revised and new side-effects recognized. For these reasons the reader is strongly urged to consult the drug companies' printed instructions before administering any of the drugs recommended in this book.

British Library Cataloguing in Publication Data
A catalogue record for this book is available from the British Library

Library of Congress Cataloging-in-Publication Data
A catalog record for this book is available from the Library of Congress

ISBN-13   978 0 340 983 546
ISBN-13 [ISE]   978 1 444 122 312 (International Students' Edition, restricted territorial availability)

1 2 3 4 5 6 7 8 9 10

Commissioning Editor: Joanna Koster
Project Editor: Sarah Penny
Production Controller: Jonathan Williams
Cover Designer: Amina Dudhia

Cover image © Sovereign, Ism/Science Photo Library

Typeset in 9.5 on 12pt Minion by Phoenix Photosetting, Chatham, Kent
Printed in India

What do you think about this book? Or any other Hodder Arnold title?
Please visit our website: www.hodderarnold.com

The editors would like to acknowledge the excellent contributions of additional authors
Carolyn Ford, Kirsty Munro, Nisha Krishnan and Sameer Umranikar,
who are not Ten Teachers but without whose significant help
this volume would not have been completed.

*I would like to thank my wife Susan and my girls Madeleine and Betsy
for their constant support and Jan, my secretary.* (AM)

*I would like to acknowledge my wife Jenny and children Harry, Anna and Ellie
for their support and love.* (SD)

Instructions for the Companion Website

This book has a companion website available at:
http://www.hodderplus.com/obsgynaebytenteachers

To access the image library included on the website, please register using the following access details:

Serial number: srfp326lw7ty

Once you have registered, you will not need a serial number but can log in using the username and password that you will create during your registration.

Contents

The Ten Teachers

Susan Bewley MB BS MD FRCOG MA (LAW AND ETHICS)

Consultant Obstetrician, Guy's and St Thomas' NHS Foundation Trust and Honorary Senior Lecturer, Kings College London, UK

Ying Cheong MB CHB BAO MA MD MRCOG

Senior Lecturer and Honorary Consultant in Obstetrics and Gynaecology; Clinical Director, Complete Fertility Centre, Southampton, UK

Sarah M Creighton MD FRCOG

Consultant Gynaecologist, University College Hospital, London, UK

Stephen Dobbs MD FRCOG

Consultant Gynaecological Oncologist, Belfast City Hospital, Belfast Trust, UK

Ailsa E Gebbie MB CHB FRCOG FFSRH DCH

Consultant in Community Gynaecology, NHS Lothian Family Planning Services, Edinburgh, UK

Janesh Gupta MSc MD FRCOG

Professor of Obstetrics and Gynaecology, University of Birmingham, Birmingham Women's Hospital, Birmingham, UK

Timothy Hillard DM FFSRH FRCOG

Consultant Obstetrician and Gynaecologist, Poole Hospital NHS Foundation Trust, Poole, UK

Andrew Horne PHD MRCOG

Senior Lecturer and Consultant Gynaecologist, University of Edinburgh, Centre for Reproductive Biology, Queen's Medical Research Institute, Edinburgh, UK

Ash Monga BMED (SCI) BM BS MRCOG

Consultant Gynaecologist, Princess Anne Hospital, Southampton University Hospital NHS Trust, Southampton, UK

David Nunns MD FRCOG

Consultant Gynaecological Oncologist, Nottingham City Hospital, Nottingham, UK

Commonly Used Abbreviations

βHCG	β-human chorionic gonadotrophin
AFP	α fetoprotein
AMH	anti-Mullerian hormone
AUC	area under the curve
BEO	bleeding of endometrial origin
BEP	bleomycin and etoposide
BMI	body mass index
BNF	British National Formulary
BRCA	breast ovarian cancer syndrome
CAIS	complete androgen insensitivity syndrome
CBAVD	congenital bilateral absence of the vas deferens
CBT	cognitive-behavioural therapy
CC	clomifene citrate
CCVR	combined contraceptive vaginal ring
CEE	conjugated equine oestrogen
CF	cystic fibrosis
CHD	coronary heart disease
CIN	cervical intraepithelial neoplasia
COC	combined oral contraception
CT	computed tomography
D&E	dilatation of the cervix and evacuation of the uterus
DHT	dihydrotestosterone
DI	donor insemination
DOA	detrusor overactivity
DSD	disorders of sex development
DUB	dysfunctional uterine bleeding
EC	emergency contraception
ED	every day
EE	ethinyl estradiol
EGF	epidermal growth factor
EOC	epithelial ovarian cancer
ERPC	evacuation of products of conception
ESR	erythrocyte sedimentation rate
ESS	endometrial stromal sarcomas
FBC	full blood count
FGF	fibroblast growth factor
FGM	female genital mutilation
FSH	follicle-stimulating hormone
GFR	glomerular filtration rate
GnRH	gonadotrophin-releasing hormone
GTD	gestational trophoblastic disorder
GUM	genitourinary medicine
HDR	high dose radiotherapy
HIV	human immunodeficiency virus
HMB	heavy menstrual bleeding
HNPCC	hereditary non-polyposis colorectal cancer syndrome
HPO	hypothalamic-pituitary-ovarian
HPV	human papilloma virus
HRT	hormone replacement therapy
HSG	hysterosalpingogram
HyCoSy	hysterocontrast synography
ICSI	intracytoplasmic sperm injection
IGFBP	insulin-like growth factor binding proteins
IMB	intermenstrual bleeding
IUI	intrauterine insemination
IUS	intrauterine system
IVF	in vitro fertilization
LAM	lactational amenorrhoea method
LARC	long-acting reversible contraception
LAVH	laparoscopy-assisted vaginal hysterectomy
LH	luteinizing hormone
LLETZ	large loop excision of transformation zone
LNG-IUS	levonorgestrel intrauterine systems
LOD	laparoscopic ovarian drilling
MBL	menstrual blood loss
MDT	multidisciplinary team
MRI	magnetic resonance imaging
MVA	manual vacuation aspiration
NAATs	nucleic acid amplification tests
NSAID	non-steroidal anti-inflammatory drug
OAB	overactive bladder
OHSS	ovarian hyperstimulation syndrome
OI	ovulation induction
PAF	platelet activating factor
PCOS	polycystic ovarian syndrome
PID	pelvic inflammatory disease
PMB	post-menopausal bleeding
PMS	premenstrual syndrome
POF	premature ovarian failure
POP	progestogen-only pill; pelvic organ prolapse
PPC	primary peritoneal carcinoma
RCOG	Royal College of Obstetricians and Gynaecologists
RMI	risk of malignancy index
SCJ	squamocolumnar junction
SERM	selective oestrogen receptor modulator

SLN	sentinel lymph node	UAE	uterine artery embolization
SSR	surgical sperm retrieval	USI	urodynamic stress incontinence
SSRIs	selective serotonin reuptake inhibitors	USS	ultrasound scan
		UTI	urinary tract infection
STI	sexually transmitted infection	VAIN	vaginal intraepithelial neoplasia
TGF	transforming growth factors	VCU	videocystourethrography
TLH	total laparoscopic hysterectomy	VEGF	vascular endothelial growth factor
TSH	thyroid stimulating hormone	VIN	vulval intraepitheial neoplasia
TVS	transvaginal ultrasound scan	VTE	venous thromboembolism
TVT	tension-free vaginal tape	WHO	World Health Organization
TZ	transformation zone		

THE GYNAECOLOGICAL HISTORY AND EXAMINATION

OVERVIEW

A careful and detailed history is essential before the examination of any patient. In addition to a good general history, focusing on the history of the presenting complaint will allow you to customize the examination to elicit the appropriate signs and make an accurate diagnosis. The gynaecological examination should always be conducted with appropriate privacy and sensitivity with a chaperone present.

History

The consultation should ideally be held in a closed room with adequate facilities and privacy. Many women will feel anxious or apprehensive about the forthcoming consultation, so it is important that the examiner establishes initial rapport with the patient and puts them at ease. The examiner should be introduced by name (a handshake often helps) and should check the patient's details. Ideally, there should be no more than one other person in the room, but any student or attending nurse should be introduced by name and their role briefly explained.

A number of women attend with their partner or close family member or friend. Provided the patient herself consents to this, there is no reason to exclude them from the initial consultation, but this should be limited to one person. In some instances, the additional person may be required to be a key part of the consultation, i.e. if there is a language or comprehension difficulty. However, it is important to recognize that some women may feel obliged to have their mother/partner present and may not provide all the relevant information with them present. At least some part of the consultation or examination should be with the woman alone to allow her to answer any specific queries more openly.

It is important to be aware of the different attitudes to various women's health issues in a religious and culturally diverse population. Appropriate respect and sensitivity should always be shown.

Enough time should be allowed for the patient to express herself and the doctor's manner should be one of interest and understanding, while guiding her with appropriate questioning. A history that is taken with sensitivity will often encourage the patient to reveal more details which may be relevant to future management.

A set template should be used for history taking, as this prevents the omission of important points and will help direct the consultation. A sample template is given below.

Symptoms

General

- Name, age and occupation
- A brief statement of the general nature and duration of the main complaints (try to use the patient's own words rather than medical terms at this stage)

History of presenting complaint

This section should focus on the presenting complaint, e.g. menstrual problems, pain, subfertility, urinary incontinence, etc. The detailed questions relating to each complaint are covered in more detail in the relevant chapters, but there are certain important aspects of a gynaecological history that should always be enquired about.

Menstrual history

- Age of menarche
- Usual duration of each period and length of cycle (usually written as mean number of days of bleeding over usual length of full cycle, e.g. 5/28)
- First day of the last period
- Pattern of bleeding: regular or irregular and length of cycle
- Amount of blood loss: more or less than usual, number of sanitary towels or tampons used, passage of clots or flooding
- Any intermenstrual or post-coital bleeding
- Any pain relating to the period, its severity and timing of onset
- Any medication taken during the period (including over-the-counter preparations).

Pelvic pain

- Site of pain, its nature and severity
- Anything that aggravates or relieves the pain – specifically enquire about relationship to menstrual cycle and intercourse
- Does the pain radiate anywhere or is it associated with bowel or bladder function (menstrual pain often radiates through to the sacral area of the back and down the thighs)?

Vaginal discharge

- Amount, colour, odour, presence of blood
- Relationship to the menstrual cycle
- Any history of sexually transmitted diseases (STDs) or recent tests
- Any vaginal dryness (post-menopausal).

Cervical screening

- Date of last smear and any previous abnormalities.

Sexual and contraceptive history

- The type of contraception used and any problems with it
- Establish whether the patient is sexually active and whether there are any difficulties or pain during intercourse.

Menopause (where relevant)

- Date of last period
- Any post-menopausal bleeding
- Any menopausal symptoms.

Previous gynaecological history

This section should include any previous gynaecological treatments or surgery.

Previous obstetric history

- Number of children with ages and birth weights.
- Any abnormalities with pregnancy, labour or the puerperium
- Number of miscarriages and gestation at which they occurred
- Any terminations of pregnancy with record of gestational age and any complications.

Previous medical history

- Any serious illnesses or operations with dates
- Family history.

Enquiry about other systems

- Appetite, weight loss, weight gain
- Bowel function (if urogynaecological complaint, more detail may be required)
- Bladder function (if urogynaecological complaint, more detail may be required).
- Enquiry of other systems.

Social history

Sensitive enquiry should be made about the woman's social situation including details of her occupation, who she lives with, her housing and whether or not she's in a stable relationship. A history regarding smoking and alcohol intake should also be obtained. Any pertinent family or other relevant social problems should be briefly discussed. If admission and surgery are being contemplated it's necessary to establish what support she has at home, particularly if she is elderly or frail.

Summary

The history should be summarized in one to two sentences before proceeding to the examination to focus the problem and alert the examiner to the salient features.

Examination

Important information about the patient can be obtained on watching them walk into the examination room. Poor mobility may affect decisions regarding surgery or future management.

Any examination should always be carried out with the patient's consent and with appropriate privacy and sensitivity. Ideally, a chaperone should be present throughout the examination.

A general examination should always be performed initially which should include examining the hands and mucous membranes for evidence of anaemia. The supraclavicular area should be palpated for the presence of nodes, particularly on the left side where in cases of abdominal malignancy one might palpate the enlarged Virchow's node (this is also known as Troissier's sign). The thyroid gland should be palpated. The chest and breasts should always be examined as part of a full examination; this is particularly relevant if there is a suspected ovarian mass, as there may be a breast tumour with secondaries of the ovaries known as Krukenburg tumours. In addition, a pleural effusion may be elicited as a consequence of abdominal ascites. A general neurological assessment should be performed, but more specific testing should be limited to cases where there is a suspicion of underlying neurological problems. The next step should be to proceed to abdominal and pelvic examination.

Abdominal examination

The patient should empty her bladder before the abdominal examination.

The patient should be comfortable and lying semi-recumbent with a sheet covering her from the

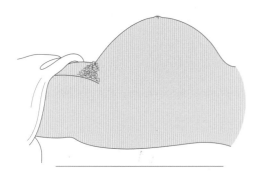

Figure 1.1   A patient in the correct position for abdominal examination showing obvious abdominal distension.

waist down, but the area from the xiphisternum to the symphysis pubis should be left exposed (Figure 1.1). It is usual to examine the women from her right hand side. Abdominal examination comprises inspection, palpation, percussion and, if appropriate, auscultation.

Inspection

The contour of the abdomen should be inspected and noted. There may be an obvious distension or mass. The presence of surgical scars, dilated veins or striae gravidarum (stretch marks) should be noted. It is important specifically to examine the umbilicus for laparoscopy scars and just above the symphysis pubis for Pfannenstiel scars (used for Caesarean section, hysterectomy, etc.). The patient should be asked to raise her head or cough and any hernias or divarication of the rectus muscles will be evident.

Palpation

First, if the patient has any abdominal pain she should be asked to point to the site – the area should not be examined until the end of palpation. Palpation using the right hand is performed examining the left lower quadrant and proceeding in a total of four steps to the right lower quadrant of the abdomen. Palpation should include examination for masses, the liver, spleen and kidneys. If a mass is present but one can palpate below it, then it is more likely to be an abdominal mass rather than a pelvic mass. It is important to remember that one of the characteristics of pelvic mass is that one cannot palpate below it. If the patient has pain her abdomen should be palpated gently and the examiner should look for signs of peritonism, i.e. guarding and rebound tenderness. The patient should also be examined for inguinal hernias and lymph nodes.

Percussion

Percussion is particularly useful if free fluid is suspected. In the recumbent position, ascitic fluid will settle down into a horseshoe shape and dullness is the flanks can be demonstrated.

As the patient moves over to her side, the dullness will move to her lowermost side. This is known as 'shifting dullness'. A fluid thrill can also be elicited. An enlarged bladder due to urinary retention will also be dull to percussion and this should be demonstrated to the examiner (many pelvic masses have disappeared after catheterization!).

Auscultation

This method is not specifically useful for the gynaecological examination. However, a patient will sometimes present with acute abdomen with bowel obstruction or a postoperative patient with ileus, and therefore listening for bowel sounds may be appropriate.

Pelvic examination

Before proceeding to a vaginal examination, the patient's verbal consent should be obtained and a female chaperone should be present for any intimate examination. Unless the patient's complaint is of urinary incontinence, it is preferable for the patient to empty her bladder before the examination. If a urine infection is suspected, a midstream sample should be collected at this point. It should go without saying that the examiner should wear gloves for this part of the procedure. There are three components to the pelvic examination.

Inspection

The external genitalia and surrounding skin, including the peri-anal area, are first inspected under a good light with the patient in the dorsal position, the hips flexed and abducted and knees flexed. The left lateral position can also be used (see below). The patient is asked to strain down to enable detection of any prolapse and also to cough, as this may show the sign of stress incontinence.

Speculum

A speculum is an instrument which is inserted into the vagina to obtain a clearer view of part of the vagina or pelvic organs. There are two principal types in widespread use. The first is a bi-valve or Cusco's speculum (Figure 1.2a), which holds back the anterior and posterior walls of the vagina and allows visualization of the cervix when opened out (Figure 1.2b). It has a retaining screw that can be tightened to allow the speculum to stay in place while a procedure or sample is taken from the cervix, e.g. smear or swab. A Sim's speculum (Figure 1.3a) is used in the left lateral position (Figure 1.3b). This is particularly useful for examination of prolapse as it allows inspection of the vaginal walls. The choice of speculum will depend on the patient's presenting problem.

Increasingly, plastic disposable speculums are being used, but if it is a metal one it is usual to warm the speculum to make the examination more comfortable for the patient. Excessive lubrication should be avoided and if a smear is being taken, lubrication with anything other than water should be avoided.

Bimanual examination

This is usually performed after the speculum examination and is performed to assess the pelvic organs. It is a technique that requires practice. There are a variety of 'model pelvises' which can be used to train the student in the basics of the examination.

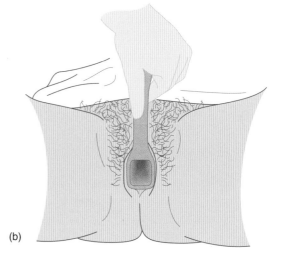

(a)   (b)

Figure 1.2   (a) Cusco's speculum; (b) Cusco's speculum in position. The speculum should be inserted at about 45° to the vertical and rotated to the vertical as it is introduced. Once it is fully inserted, the blades should be opened up to visualize the cervix.

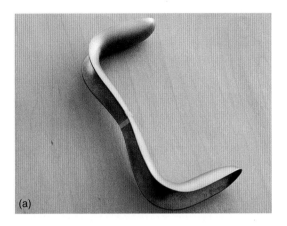

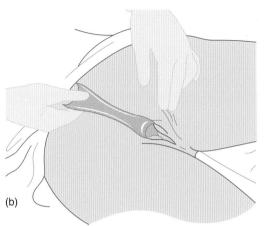

Figure 1.3 (a) Sim's speculum; (b) Sim's speculum inserted with the patient in the left lateral position. The speculum is being used to hold back the posterior vaginal walls to allow inspection of the anterior wall and vault. The speculum can be rotated 180° or withdrawn slowly to visualize the posterior wall.

Some universities are now utilizing gynaecology teaching assistants who are paid volunteers who allow themselves to be examined and will talk the student through the examination. It is customary to use the left hand to part the labia and expose the vestibule and then insert one or two fingers of the right hand into the vagina. The fingers are passed upwards and backwards to reach the cervix (Figure 1.4a). The cervix is palpated and any irregularity, hardness or tenderness noted. The left hand is now placed on the abdomen below the umbilicus and pressed down into the pelvis to palpate the fundus of the uterus. The size, shape, position, mobility, consistency and tenderness are noted. The normal uterus is pear-shaped and about 9 cm in length. It is usually anterior

(antiverted) or posterior (retroverted) and freely mobile and non-tender. The tips of the fingers are then placed into each lateral fornix to palpate the adenexae (tubes and ovaries) on each side. The fingers are pushed backwards and upwards, while at the same time pushing down in the corresponding area with the fingers of the abdominal hand (Figure 1.4b). It is unusual to be able to feel normal ovaries, except in very thin women. Any swelling or tenderness is noted, although remember that normal ovaries can be very tender when directly palpated. The posterior fornix should also be palpated to identify the uterosacral ligaments which may be tender or scarred in women with endometriosis.

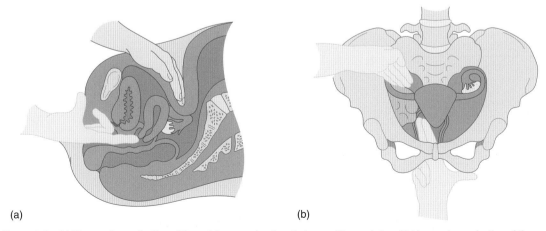

(a)   (b)

Figure 1.4 (a) Bimanual examination of the pelvis assessing the uterine position and size; (b) bimanual examination of the lateral fornix.

Rectal examination

A rectal examination can be used as an alternative to a vaginal examination in children and in adults who have never had sex. It is less sensitive than a vaginal examination and can be quite uncomfortable, but it will help pick up a pelvic mass. In some situations, a rectal examination can also be useful as well as a vaginal examination to differentiate between an enterocele and a rectocele or to palpate the uterosacral ligaments more thoroughly. Occasionally, a rectovaginal examination (index finger in the vagina and middle finger in the rectum) may be useful to identify a lesion in the rectovaginal septum.

Investigations

Once the examination is complete, the patient should be given the opportunity to dress in privacy and come back into the consultation room to sit down and discuss the findings. You should now be able to give a summary of the whole case and formulate a differential diagnosis. This will then determine the appropriate further investigations (if any) that should be needed. Swabs and smears should be taken at the time of the examination and a midstream specimen of urine (MSU) when the patient empties her bladder before the examination. The need for further investigations, such as ultrasound, colposcopy and urodynamics, is discussed in the relevant chapters.

Key Points

- The consultation should be performed in a private environment and in a sensitive fashion
- The examiner should introduce him/herself, be courteous and explain what is about to happen and why.
- The examiner should be familiar with the history template and use it regularly to avoid omissions.
- Remember to summarize the history before proceeding to the examination.
- A chaperone should always be present for an intimate examination.
- The examiner should be sensitive to the patient's needs and anxiety and respect her privacy and dignity.
- The examination should always begin with a general assessment of the patient.
- The patient should be asked to inform the examiner if the examination is uncomfortable.
- The examiner should reassure the patient during the examination and give feedback about what is being done.
- After the examination, the examiner should make sure that the patient is comfortable and allow her to get dressed in privacy.
- The examiner should explain the findings to the patient in suitable language and give her the opportunity to ask questions.
- Prepare a differential diagnosis and order any appropriate investigations.

OVERVIEW

A good understanding of the embryological development and resulting genital anatomy is essential. This is particularly important with respect to the congenital anomalies described in Chapter 3, but also underpins basic understanding of the impact of all gynaecological disease processes.

Embryology

The normal early pregnancy

Implantation and subsequent placental development in the human require complex adaptive changes of the uterine wall constituents.

Development of the blastocyst

At the beginning of the 4th week after the last menstrual period, the implanted blastocyst is composed, from outside to inside, of the trophoblastic ring, the extra-embryonic mesoderm and the amniotic cavity and the primary yolk sac, separated by the bilaminar embryonic disk. The extra-embryonic mesoderm progressively increases, and 12 days after ovulation (around the 26th menstrual day) it contains isolated spaces that rapidly fuse to form the extra-embryonic coelom. As the latter forms, the primary yolk sac decreases in size and the secondary yolk sac arises from cells growing from the embryonic disk inside the primary yolk sac.

Formation of the placenta

Primary chorionic villi develop between 13 and 15 days after ovulation (end of 4th week of gestation). Simultaneously, blood vessels start to develop in the extra-embryonic mesoderm of the yolk sac, the connecting stalk and the chorion. The primary villi are composed of a central mass of cytotrophoblast surrounded by a thick layer of syncytiotrophoblast.

During the 5th week of gestation, they acquire a central mesenchymal core from the extra-embryonic mesoderm and become branched, forming the secondary villi. The appearance of embryonic blood vessels within their mesenchymal cores transformsthe secondary villi into tertiary villi. Up to 10 weeks' gestation, which corresponds to the last week of the embryonic period (stages 19 to 23), villi cover the entire surface of the chorionic sac.

As the gestational sac grows during fetal life, the villi associated with the decidua capsularis surrounding the amniotic sac become compressed and degenerate, forming an avascular shell known as the chorion laeve, or smooth chorion. Conversely, the villi associated with the decidua basalis proliferate, forming the chorion frondosum or definitive placenta.

Normal placentation

As soon as the blastocyst has hatched, the tropho-ectoderm layer attaches to the cell surface of the endometrium and, by simple displacement, early trophoblastic penetration within the endometrial stroma occurs. Progressively, the entire blastocyst will sink into maternal decidua and the migrating trophoblastic cells will encounter venous channels of increasing size, then superficial arterioles and, during the 4th week, the spiral arteries. The trophoblastic cells infiltrate deep into the decidua and reach the deciduo-myometrial junction at between 8 and 12 weeks' gestation. This extravillous trophoblast penetrates the inner third of the myometrium via the interstitial ground substance and affects its mechanical and electrophysiological properties by increasing its expansile capacity. The trophoblastic infiltration of the myometrium is progressive and achieved before 18 weeks' gestation in normal pregnancies.

Ultrasound imaging

The gestational sac representing the deciduo-placental interface and the chorionic cavity are the first sonographic evidence of a pregnancy. The gestational sac can be visualized with transvaginal ultrasound around 4.4–4.6 weeks (32–34 days) following the onset of the last menstruation, when it reaches a size of 2–4 mm. By contrast, the gestational sac can only be observed by means of abdominal ultrasound imaging during the 5th week post-menstruation.

The first embryonic structure that becomes visible inside the chorionic cavity is the secondary yolk sac, when the gestational sac reaches 8 mm. Demonstration of the yolk sac reliably indicates that an intrauterine fluid collection represents a true gestational sac, thus excluding the possibility of a pseudosac or an ectopic pregnancy.

Symptomatology

The classical symptom triad for early pregnancy disorders is amenorrhoea, pelvic or low abdominal pain and vaginal bleeding. Pregnancy symptoms are often non-specific and many women of reproductive age have irregular menstrual cycles. The first test to confirm the existence of pregnancy is for the detection of human chorionic gonadotrophin (hCG) in the patient's urine or plasma.

Pregnancy tests

Human chorionic gonadotrophin is a placental-derived glycoprotein, composed of two subunits, alpha and beta, which maintains the corpus luteum for the first 7 weeks of gestation. Extremely small quantities of hCG are produced by the pituitary gland and thus plasma hCG is almost exclusively produced by the placenta. Human chorionic gonadotrophin has a half-life of 6–24 hours and rises to a peak in pregnancy at 9–11 weeks' gestation.

Urine testing

It is possible to detect low levels of hCG in urine by rapid (1–2 min) dipstick tests. The sensitivity of these tests is high (detection limit of around 50iu/L) and they produce positive results around 14 days after ovulation.

Plasma testing

Measurement of hCG in plasma is more accurate (detection limit around 0.1–0.3iu/L) and is able to detect a pregnancy 6–7 days after ovulation, which corresponds to the time of implantation. Measurement of hCG levels may help to diagnose ectopic pregnancy and is of pivotal importance in the follow-up of some pregnancy disorders.

The mechanism of sex differentiation into a female or male fetus is described in Chapter 3. Once the gonad has become an ovary, subsequent female development follows.

The ovary

At approximately 4–5 weeks of embryonic life, genital ridges are formed overlying the embryonic kidney. At this stage, these are identical in both sexes. The primitive gonad is formed between 5 and 7 weeks of gestation, when undifferentiated germ cells migrate from the yolk sac to the genital ridges. In the absence of male determinants, the primitive gonad becomes an ovary. Granulosa cells derived from the proliferating coelomic epithelium surround the germ cells and form primordial follicles. Each primordial follicle consists of an oocyte within a single layer of granulosa cells. Theca cells develop from the proliferating coelomic epithelium and are separated from the granulosa cells by a basal lamina. The maximum number of primordial follicles is reached at 20 weeks gestation when at this time there are six to seven million primordial follicles present. The numbers of these reduce by atresia and by birth one to two million are present. Atresia continues throughout childhood and by menstruation 300 000 to 400 000 are present.

The development of an oocyte within a primordial follicle is arrested at the prophase of its first meiotic division. It remains in that state until it regresses or enters the meiotic process shortly before ovulation.

The uterus and vagina

The genital system develops in close association with the urinary system. During the fifth week of embryonic life, the nephrogenic duct develops from the mesoderm and forms the urogenital ridge and mesonephric duct (Figure 2.1). The mesonephric duct (also named the Wolffian duct) develops under the influence of testosterone into vas deferens,

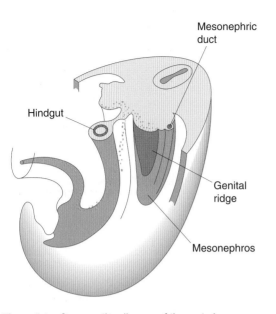

Figure 2.1   Cross section diagram of the posterior abdominal wall showing genital ridge.

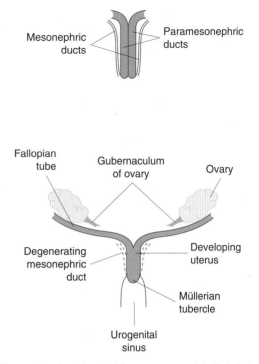

Figure 2.2   Caudal part of the paramesonephric duct (top) fusion to form uterus and Fallopian tubes.

epididymus and seminal vesicle. In the female fetus, the Wolffian system regresses. The female reproductive tracts develop from paired ducts which are adjacent to the mesonephric duct and so are called the paramesonephric ducts (or Mullerian ducts). These extend caudally to project into the posterior wall of the urogenital sinus as the Mullerian tubercle. These fuse in the midline distally to form the uterus, cervix and proximal two thirds of the vagina. The unfused caudal segments form the Fallopian tubes. The distal vagina is formed from the sinovaginal bulbs in the upper portion of the urogenital sinus (Figure 2.2).

The external genitalia

Between the fifth and seventh weeks of life, the cloacal folds which are a pair of swellings adjacent to the cloacal membrane fuse anteriorly to become the genital tubercle. This will become the clitoris. The perineum develops and divides the cloaca membrane into an anterior urogenital membrane and a posterior anal membrane. The cloacal folds anteriorly are called the urethral folds which form the labia minora. Another pair of folds within the cloacal membrane form the labioscrotal folds which eventually become the labia majora. The urogenital sinus becomes the vestibule of the vagina. The external genitalia are recognizably female by the end of 12 weeks gestation.

Anatomy

The external genitalia

The external genitalia is commonly called the vulva and includes the mons pubis, labia majora and minora, the vaginal vestibule, the clitoris and the greater vestibular glands (Figure 2.3). The mons pubis is a fibro-fatty pad covered by hair-bearing skin which covers the body of the pubic bones.

The labia majora are two folds of skin with underlying adipose tissue lying either side of the vagina opening. They contain sebaceous and sweat glands and a few specialized apocrine glands. In the deepest part of each labium is a core of fatty tissue continuous with that of the inguinal canal and the fibres of the round ligament terminate here.

The labia minora are two thin folds of skin that lie between the labia majora. These vary in size and may protrude beyond the labia major where they are visible, but may also be concealed by the labia majora. Anteriorly, they divide in two to form the prepuce and frenulum of the clitoris (clitoral hood). Posteriorly,

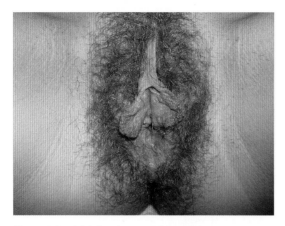

Figure 2.3   Adult female external genitalia.

they divide to form a fold of skin called the fourchette at the back of the vagina introitus. They contain sebaceous glands, but have no adipose tissue. They are not well developed before puberty and atrophy after the menopause. Both the labia minora and labia majora become engorged during sexual arousal.

The clitoris is an erectile structure measuring approximately 0.5–3.5 cm in length. The body of the clitoris is the main part of the visible clitoris and is made up of paired columns of erectile tissue and vascular tissue called the 'corpora cavernosa'. These become the crura at the bottom of the clitoris and run deeper and laterally. The vestibule is the cleft between the labia minora. It contains openings of the urethra, the Bartholin's glands and the vagina. The vagina is surrounded by two bulbs of erectile and vascular tissue which are extensive and almost completely cover the distal vaginal wall. These have traditionally been named the bulb of the vaginal vestibule, although recent work on both dissection and magnetic resonance imaging (MRI) suggests that they may be part of the clitoris and should be renamed 'clitoral bulbs'. Their function is unknown but they probably add support to the distal vaginal wall to enhance its rigidity during penetration.

The Bartholin's glands are bilateral and about the size of a pea. They open via a 2-cm duct into the vestibule below the hymen and contribute to lubrication during intercourse.

The hymen is a thin covering of mucous membrane across the entrance to the vagina. It is usually perforated which allows menstruation. The hymen is ruptured during intercourse and any remaining tags are called 'carunculae myrtiformes'.

In the prepubertal vulva, no hair is present and there is little adipose deposition. During puberty, pubic hair develops and fat deposition within the labia gives a more womanly shape. After the menopause, with the fall in oestrogen levels, the labia minora lose fat and become thinner, but may become elongated. The vaginal opening becomes smaller.

The internal reproductive organs

The vagina

The vagina is a fibromuscular canal lined with stratified squamous epithelium that leads from the uterus to the vulva (Figure 2.4). It is longer in the posterior wall (approximately 9 cm) than in the anterior wall (approximately 7 cm). The vaginal walls are normally in apposition, except at the vault where they are separated by the cervix. The vault of the vagina is divided into four fornices: posterior, anterior and two lateral.

The mid-vagina is a transverse slit while the lower vagina is an H-shape in transverse section. The vaginal walls are lined with transverse folds. The vagina has no glands and is kept moist by secretions from the uterine and cervical glands and by transudation from its epithelial lining. The epithelium is thick and rich in glycogen which increases in the post-ovulatory phase of the cycle. However, before puberty and after the menopause, the vagina is devoid of glycogen due to the lack of oestrogen. Doderlein's bacillus is a normal commensal of the vaginal flora and breaks down glycogen to form lactic acid and producing a pH of around 4.5. This has a protective role for the vagina in decreasing the growth of pathogenic bacteria.

The upper posterior wall forms the anterior peritoneal reflection of the pouch of Douglas. The middle third is separated from the rectum by pelvic fascia and the lower third abuts the perineal body. Anteriorly, the vagina is in direct contact with the base of the bladder, while the urethra runs down the lower half in the midline to open into the vestibule. Its muscles fuse with the anterior vagina wall. Laterally, at the fornices, the vagina is related to the cardinal ligaments. Below this are the levator ani muscles and the ischiorectal fossae. The cardinal ligaments and the uterosacral ligaments which form

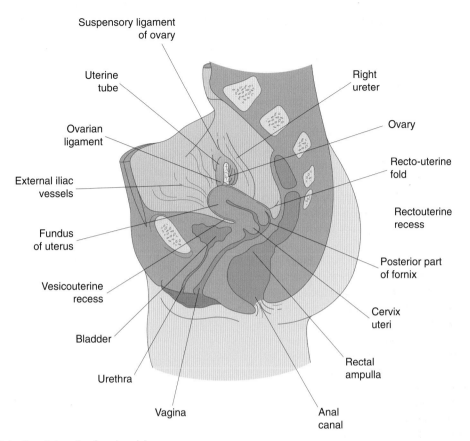

Suspensory ligament
of ovary

Uterine
tube

Ovarian
ligament

External iliac
vessels

Fundus
of uterus

Vesicouterine
recess

Bladder

Urethra

Vagina

Right
ureter

Ovary

Recto-uterine
fold

Rectouterine
recess

Posterior part
of fornix

Cervix
uteri

Rectal
ampulla

Anal
canal

Figure 2.4 Saggital section female pelvis.

posteriorly from the parametrium support the upper part of the vagina.

At birth, the vagina is under the influence of maternal oestrogens so the epithelium is well developed. After a couple of weeks, the effects of the oestrogen disappear and the pH rises to 7 and the epithelium atrophies. At puberty, the reverse occurs and finally at the menopause the vagina tends to shrink and the epithelium atrophies.

The uterus

The uterus is shaped like an inverted pear tapering inferiorly to the cervix and in its non-pregnant state is situated entirely within the pelvis. It is hollow and has thick, muscular walls. Its maximum external dimensions are approximately 7.5 cm long, 5 cm wide and 3 cm thick. An adult uterus weighs approximately 70 g. In the upper part, the uterus is termed the body or 'corpus'. The area of insertion of each Fallopian tube is termed the 'cornu' and that part of the body

above the cornu is called the 'fundus'. The uterus tapers to a small constricted area, the isthmus, and below this is the cervix which projects obliquely into the vagina. The longitudinal axis of the uterus is approximately at right angles to the vagina and normally tilts forward. This is called 'anteversion'. In addition, the long axis of the cervix is rarely the same as the long axis of the uterus. The uterus is also usually flexed forward on itself at the isthmus – antiflexion. However, in around 20 per cent of women, the uterus is tilted backwards – retroversion and retroflexion. This has no pathological significance.

The cavity of the uterus is the shape of an inverted triangle and when sectioned coronally the Fallopian tubes open at lateral angles The constriction at the isthmus where the corpus joins the cervix is the anatomical os. Seen microscopically, the site of the histological internal os is where the mucous membrane of the isthmus becomes that of the cervix.

The uterus consists of three layers: the outer serous layer (peritoneum), the middle muscular layer (myometrium) and the inner mucous layer (endometrium). The peritoneum covers the body of the uterus and posteriorly the supravaginal part of the cervix. The peritoneum is intimately attached to a subserous fibrous layer, except laterally where it spreads out to form the leaves of the broad ligament.

The muscular myometrium forms the main bulk of the uterus and is made up of interlacing smooth muscle fibres intermingling with areolar tissue, blood vessels, nerves and lymphatics. Externally, these are mostly longitudinal, but the larger intermediate layer has interlacing longitudinal, oblique and transverse fibres. Internally, they are mainly longitudinal and circular.

The inner endometrial layer has tubular glands that dip into the myometrium. The endometrial layer is covered by a single layer of columnar epithelium. Ciliated prior to puberty, this epithelium is mostly lost due to the effects of pregnancy and menstruation. The endometrium undergoes cyclical changes during menstruation and varies in thickness between 1 and 5 mm.

The cervix

The cervix is narrower than the body of the uterus and is approximately 2.5 cm in length. Lateral to the cervix lies cellular connective tissue called the parametrium. The ureter runs about 1 cm laterally to the supravaginal cervix within the parametrium. The posterior aspect of the cervix is covered by the peritoneum of the pouch of Douglas.

The upper part of the cervix mostly consists of involuntary muscle, whereas the lower part is mainly fibrous connective tissue. The mucous membrane of the cervical canal (endocervix) has anterior and posterior columns from which folds radiate out, the 'arbour vitae'. It has numerous deep glandular follicles that secrete clear alkaline mucus, the main component of physiological vaginal discharge. The epithelium of the endocervix is columnar and is also ciliated in its upper two thirds. This changes to stratified squamous epithelium around the region of the external os and the junction of these two types of epithelium is called the 'squamocolumnar junction' or transformation zone. This is an area of rapid cell division and approximately 90 per cent of cervical cancers arise here.

Age changes

The disappearance of maternal oestrogens from the circulation after birth causes the uterus to decrease in length by around one third and in weight by around one half. The cervix is then twice the length of the uterus. During childhood, the uterus grows slowly in length, in parallel with height and age. The average longitudinal diameter ranges from 2.5 cm at the age of two years, to 3.5 cm at ten years. After the onset of puberty, the anteroposterior and transverse diameters of the uterus start to increase leading to a sharper rise in the volume of the uterus. The increase in uterine volume continues well after menarche and the uterus reaches its adult size and configuration by the late teenage years. After the menopause, the uterus atrophies, the mucosa becomes very thin, the glands almost disappear and the wall becomes relatively less muscular.

The Fallopian tubes

The Fallopian tube extends outwards from the uterine cornu to end near the ovary. At the abdominal ostium, the tube opens into the peritoneal cavity which is therefore in communication with the exterior of the body via the uterus and the vagina. This is essential to allow the sperm and egg to meet. The Fallopian tubes convey the ovum from the ovary towards the uterus which promotes oxygenation and nutrition for sperm, ovum and zygote should fertilization occur.

The Fallopian tube runs in the upper margin of the broad ligament part of which, known as the mesosalpinx, encloses it so the tube is completely covered with peritoneum, except for a narrow strip along this inferior aspect. Each tube is about 10 cm long and is described in four parts:

1 The interstitial portion
2 The isthmus
3 The ampulla
4 The infundibulum or fimbrial portion.

The interstitial portion lies within the wall of the uterus, while the isthmus is the narrow portion adjoining the uterus. This passes into the widest and longest portion, the ampulla. This, in turn, terminates in the extremity known as the 'infundibulum'. The opening of the tube into the peritoneal cavity is surrounded by finger-like processes, known as fimbria, into which the muscle coat does not extend.

The inner surfaces of the fimbriae are covered by ciliated epithelium which is similar to the lining of the Fallopian tube itself. One of these fimbriae is longer than the others and extends to and partially embraces the ovary. The muscular fibres of the wall of the tube are arranged in an inner circular and an outer longitudinal layer.

The tubal epithelium forms a number of branched folds or plicae which run longitudinally; the lumen of the ampulla is almost filled with these folds. The folds have a cellular stroma, but at their bases the epithelium is only separated from the muscle by a very scanty amount of stroma. There is no submucosa and there are no glands. The epithelium of the Fallopian tubes contains two functioning cell types; the ciliated cells which act to produce constant current of fluid in the direction of the uterus and the secretory cells which contribute to the volume of tubal fluid. Changes occur under the influence of the menstrual cycle, but there is no cell shedding during menstruation.

The ovaries

The size and appearance of the ovaries depends on both age and stage of the menstrual cycle. In a child, the ovaries are small structures approximately 1.5 cm long; however, they increase to adult size in puberty due to proliferation of stromal cells and commencing maturation of the ovarian follicles. In the young adult, they are almond-shaped and measure approximately 3 cm long, 1.5 cm wide and 1 cm thick. After the menopause, no active follicles are present and the ovary becomes smaller with a wrinkled surface. The ovary is the only intra-abdominal structure not to be covered by peritoneum. Each ovary is attached to the cornu of the uterus by the ovarian ligament and at the hilum to the broad ligament by the mesovarium which contains its supply of nerves and blood vessels. Laterally, each ovary is attached to the suspensory ligament of the ovary with folds of peritoneum which becomes continuous with that of the overlying psoas major.

Anterior to the ovaries lie the Fallopian tubes, the superior portion of the bladder and the uterovesical pouch. It is bound behind by the ureter where it runs downwards and forwards in front of the internal iliac artery.

Structure

The ovary has a central vascular medulla consisting of loose connective tissue containing many elastin fibres and non-striated muscle cells. It has an outer thicker cortex, denser than the medulla consisting of networks of reticular fibres and fusiform cells, although there is no clear-cut demarcation between the two. The surface of the ovaries is covered by a single layer of cuboidal cells, the germinal epithelium. Beneath this is an ill-defined layer of condensed connective tissue called the 'tunica albuginea', which increases in density with age. At birth, numerous primordial follicles are found mostly in the cortex, but some are found in the medulla. With puberty, some form each month into the graafian follicles which will at a later stage of development form corpus lutea and ultimately atretic follicles, the corpora albicans.

Vestigial structures

Vestigial remains of the mesonephric duct and tubules are always present in young children, but are variable structures in adults. The epoophoron, a series of parallel blind tubules, lies in the broad ligament between the mesovarium and the Fallopian tube. The tubules run to the rudimentary duct of the epoophoron which runs parallel to the lateral Fallopian tube. Situated in the broad ligament between the epoophoron and the uterus are occasionally seen a few rudimentary tubules, the paroophoron. In a few individuals, the caudal part of the mesonephric duct is well developed running alongside the uterus to the internal os. This is the duct of Gartner.

The bladder, urethra and ureter

The bladder

The vesicle or bladder wall is made of involuntary muscle arranged in an inner longitudinal layer, a middle circular layer and an outer longitudinal layer. It is lined with transitional epithelium and has an average capacity of 400 mL.

The ureters open into the base of the bladder after running medially for about 1 cm through the vesical wall. The urethra leaves the bladder in front of the ureteric orifices. The triangular area lying between the ureteric orifices and the internal meatus of the ureter is known as the 'trigone'. At the internal meatus, the middle layer of vesical muscle forms anterior and posterior loops round the neck of the bladder, some fibres of the loops being continuous with the circular muscle of the urethra.

The base of the bladder is adjacent to the cervix, with only a thin layer of tissue intervening. It is separated from the anterior vaginal wall below by the pubocervical fascia which stretches from the pubis to the cervix.

The urethra

The female urethra is about 3.5 cm long and is lined with transitional epithelium. It has a slight posterior angulation at the junction of its lower and middle thirds. The smooth muscle of its wall is arranged in outer longitudinal and inner circular layers. As the urethra passes through the two layers of the urogenital diaphragm (triangular ligament), it is embraced by the striated fibres of the deep transverse perineal muscle (compressor urethrae) and some of the striated fibres of this muscle form a loop on the urethra. Between the muscular coat and the epithelium is a plexus of veins. There are a number of tubular mucous glands and in the lower part a number of crypts which occasionally become infected. In its upper two thirds, the urethra is separated from the symphysis by loose connective tissue, but in its lower third it is attached to the pubic ramus on each side by strong bands of fibrous tissue called the 'pubourethral tissue'. Posteriorly, it is firmly attached in its lower two thirds to the anterior vaginal wall. This means that the upper part of the urethra is mobile, but the lower part is relatively fixed.

Medial fibres of the pubococcygeus of the levator ani muscles are inserted into the urethra and vaginal wall. When they contract, they pull the anterior vaginal wall and the upper part of the urethra forwards forming an angle of about 100° between the posterior wall of the urethra and the bladder base. On voluntary voiding of urine, the base of the bladder and the upper part of the urethra descend and the posterior angle disappears so that the base of the bladder and the posterior wall of the urethra come to lie in a straight line. It was formerly claimed that absence of this posterior angle was the cause of stress incontinence, but this is probably only one of a number of mechanisms responsible.

The ureter

As the ureter crosses the pelvic brim, it lies in front of the bifurcation of the common iliac artery. It runs downwards and forwards on the lateral wall of the pelvis to reach the pelvic floor and then passes inwards and forwards attached to the peritoneum of the back of the broad ligament to pass beneath the uterine artery. It next passes forward through a fibrous tunnel, the ureteric canal, in the upper part of the cardinal ligament. Finally, it runs close to the lateral vaginal fornix to enter the trigone of the bladder.

Its blood supply is derived from small branches of the ovarian artery, from a small vessel arising near the iliac bifurcation, from a branch of the uterine artery where it crosses beneath it and from small branches of the vesical artery.

Because of is close relationship to the cervix, the vault of the vagina and the uterine artery, the ureter may be damaged during hysterectomy. Apart from being cut or tied, in radical procedures, the ureter may undergo necrosis because of interference with its blood supply. It may be displaced upwards by fibromyomata or cysts which are growing between the layers of the broad ligament and may suffer injury if its position is not noticed at operation.

The rectum

The rectum extends from the level of the third sacral vertebra to a point about 2.5 cm in front of the coccyx where it passes through the pelvic floor to become continuous with the anal canal. Its direction follows the curve of the sacrum and is about 11 cm in length. The front and sides are covered by the peritoneum of the rectovaginal pouch. In the middle third, only the front is covered by peritoneum. In the lower third, there is no peritoneal covering and the rectum is separated from the posterior wall of the vagina by the rectovaginal fascial septum. Lateral to the rectum are the uterosacral ligaments beside which run some of the lymphatics draining the cervix and vagina.

The pelvic muscles, ligaments and fascia

The pelvic diaphragm

The pelvic diaphragm is formed by the levator ani muscles which are broad, flat muscles the fibres of which pass downwards and inwards (Figure 2.5). The two muscles, one on either side, constitute the pelvic diaphragm. The muscle arises by linear origin from:

- the lower part of the body of the os pubis;
- the internal surface of the parietal pelvic fascia along the white line;
- the pelvic surface of the ischial spine.

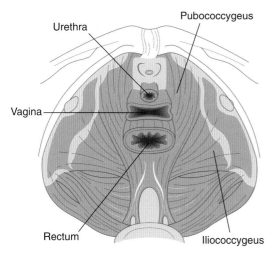

Urethra

Pubococcygeus

Vagina

Rectum

Iliococcygeus

Figure 2.5   Pelvic floor musculature.

The levator ani muscles are inserted into:

- the preanal raphe and the central point of the perineum where one muscle meets the other on the opposite side;
- the wall of the anal canal, where the fibres blend with the deep external sphincter muscle;
- the postanal or anococcygeal raphe, where again one muscle meets the other on the opposite side;
- the lower part of the coccyx.

The muscle is described in two parts:

1 The pubococcygeus which arises from the pubic bone and the anterior part of the tendinous arch of the pelvic fascia (white line)

2 The iliococcygeus which arises from the posterior part of the tendinous arch and the ischial spine.

The medial borders of the pubococcygeus muscle pass on either side from the pubic bone to the preanal raphe. They thus embrace the vagina and on contraction have some sphincteric action. The nerve supply is from the third and fourth sacral nerves. The pubococcygeus muscles support the pelvic and abdominal viscera, including the bladder. The medial edge passes beneath the bladder and runs laterally to the urethra, into which some of its fibres are inserted. Together with the fibres from the opposite muscle, they form a loop which maintains the angle between the posterior aspect of the urethra and the bladder base. During micturition, this loop relaxes to allow the bladder neck and upper urethra to open and descend.

Urogenital diaphragm

The urogenital diaphragm (triangular ligament) is made up of two layers of pelvic fascia which fill the gap between the descending pubic rami and lies beneath the levator ani muscles. The deep transverse perineal muscles (compressor urethrae) lies between the two layers and the diaphragm is pierced by the urethra and vagina.

The perineal body

This is a mass of muscular tissue that lies between the anal canal and the lower third of the vagina. Its apex is at the lower end of the rectovaginal septum at the point where the rectum and posterior vaginal walls come into contact. Its base is covered with skin and extends from the fourchette to the anus. It is the point of insertion of the superficial perineal muscles and is bounded above by the levator ani muscles where they come into contact in the midline between the posterior vaginal wall and the rectum.

The pelvic peritoneum

The peritoneum is reflected from the lateral borders of the uterus to form on either side a double fold of peritoneum – the broad ligament. Despite the name, this is not a ligament but a peritoneal fold and it does not support the uterus. The Fallopian tube runs in the upper free edge of the broad ligament as far as the point at which the tube opens into the peritoneal cavity. The part of the broad ligament that is lateral to the opening is called the 'infundibulopelvic fold' and in it the ovarian vessels and nerves pass from the side wall of the pelvis to lie between the two layers of the broad ligament. The mesosalpinx, the portion of the broad ligament which lies above the ovary is layered; between its layers are to be seen any Wolffian remnants which may remain. Below the ovary, the base of the broad ligament widens out and contains a considerable amount of loose connective tissue called the 'parametrium'. The ureter is attached to the posterior leaf of the broad ligament at this point.

The ovary is attached to the posterior layer of the broad ligament by a short mesentry (the mesovarium) through which the ovarian vessels and nerves enter the hilum.

The ovarian ligament and round ligament

The ovarian ligament lies beneath the posterior layer of the broad ligament and passes from the medial pole of the ovary to the uterus just below the point of entry of the Fallopian tube.

The round ligament is the continuation of the same structure and runs forwards under the anterior leaf of peritoneum to enter the inguinal canal ending in the subcutaneous tissue of the labium major.

The pelvic fascia and pelvic cellular tissue

Connective tissue fills the irregular spaces between the various pelvic organs. Much of it is loose cellular tissue, but in some places it is condensed to form strong ligaments which contain some smooth muscle fibres and which form the fascial sheaths which enclose the various viscera. The pelvic arteries, veins, lymphatics, nerves and ureters runs though it. The cellular tissue is continuous above with the extraperitoneal tissue of the abdominal wall, but below it is cut off from the ischiorectal fossa by the pelvic fascia and the lavatory ani muscles. The pelvic fascia may be regarded as a specialized part of this connective tissue and has parietal and visceral components.

The parietal pelvic fascia lines the wall of the pelvic cavity covering the obturator and pyramidalis muscles. There is a thickened tendinous arch (or white line) on the side wall of the pelvis. It is here that the levator ani muscle arises and the cardinal ligament gains its lateral attachment. Where the parietal pelvic fascia encounters bone, as in the pubic region, it blends with the periosteum. It also forms the upper layer of the urogenital diaphragm (triangular ligament).

Each viscus has a fascial sheath which is dense in the case of the vagina and cervix and at the base of the bladder, but is tenuous or absent over the body of the uterus and the dome of the bladder. From the point of view of the gynaecologist, certain parts of the visceral fascia are important, as follows:

- The cardinal ligaments (transverse cervical ligaments) provide the essential support of the uterus and vaginal vault. These are two strong fan-shaped fibromuscular bands which pass from the cervix and vaginal vault to the side wall of the pelvis on either side.
- The uterosacral ligaments run from the cervix and vaginal vault to the sacrum. In the erect position,

they are almost vertical in direction and support the cervix.
- The bladder is supported laterally by condensations of the vesical pelvic fascia one each side and by a sheet of pubocervical fascia which lies beneath it anteriorly.

The blood supply

Arteries supplying the pelvic organs

Because the ovary develops on the posterior abdominal wall and later migrates down into the pelvis, it carries its blood supply with it directly from the abdominal aorta. The ovarian artery arises from the aorta just below the renal artery and runs downwards on the surface of the psoas muscle to the pelvic brim, where it crosses in front of the ureter and then passes into the infundibulopelvic fold of the broad ligament (Figure 2.6). The artery divides into branches that supply the ovary and tube and then run on to reach the uterus where they anastamose with the terminal branches of the uterine artery.

The internal iliac (hypogastric) artery

This vessel is about 4 cm in length and begins at the bifurcation of the common iliac artery in front of the sacroiliac joint. It soon divides into anterior and posterior branches: the branches that supply the pelvic organs are all from the anterior division.

The uterine artery provides the main blood supply to the uterus. The artery first runs downwards on the lateral wall of the pelvis, in the same direction as the ureter. It then turns inward and forwards lying in the base of the broad ligament. On reaching the wall of the uterus, the artery turns upwards to run tortuously to the upper part of the uterus, where it anastomoses with the ovarian artery. In this part of its course, it sends many branches into the substance of the uterus. The uterine artery supplies a branch to the ureter as it crosses it and shortly afterwards another branch is given off to supply the cervix and upper vagina.

The vaginal artery is another branch of the internal iliac artery that runs at a lower level to supply the vagina. The vesical arteries are variable in numbers and supply the bladder and terminal ureter. One usually runs in the roof of the ureteric canal.

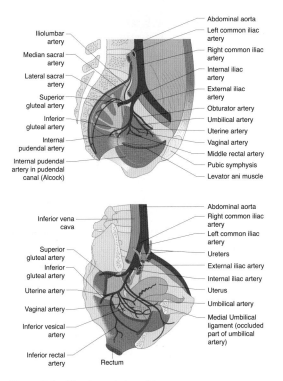

Figure 2.6   Blood supply to pelvis.

The middle rectal artery often arises in common with the lowest vesical artery.

The pudendal artery is another branch of the internal iliac artery. It leaves the pelvic cavity through the sciatic foramen and, after winding round the ischial spine, enters the ischiorectal fossa where it gives off the inferior rectal artery. It terminates in branches that supply the perineal and vulval arteries, including the erectile tissue of the vestibular bulbs and clitoris.

The superior rectal artery

This artery is the continuation of the inferior mesenteric artery and descends in the base of the mesocolon. It divides into two branches which run on either side of the rectum and supply numerous branches to it.

The pelvic veins

The veins around the bladder, uterus, vagina and rectum form plexuses which intercommunicate freely. Venous drainage from the uterine, vaginal and

vesical plexus is chiefly into the internal iliac veins. Venous drainage from the rectal plexus is via the superior rectal veins to the inferior mesenteric veins, and the middle and inferior rectal veins to the internal pudendal veins and so to the iliac veins.

The ovarian veins on each side begin in the pampiniform plexus that lies between the layers of the broad ligament. At first, there are two veins on each side accompanying the corresponding ovarian artery. Higher up the vein becomes single, with that on the right ending in the inferior vena cava and that on the left in the left renal vein.

The pelvic lymphatics

Lymph draining from all the lower extremities and the vulva and perineal regions is all filtered through the inguinal and superficial femoral nodes before continuing along the deep pathways on the side wall of the pelvis. One deep chain passes upwards lateral to the major blood vessels, forming in turn the external iliac, common iliac and para-aortic groups of nodes.

Medially, another chain of vessels passes from the deep femoral nodes through the femoral canal to the obturator and internal iliac groups of nodes. These last nodes are interspersed among the origins of the branches of the internal iliac artery receiving lymph directly from the organs supplied by this artery including the upper vagina, cervix and body of the uterus.

From the internal iliac and common iliac nodes, afferent vessels pass up the para-aortic chains and finally all lymphatic drainage from the legs and pelvis flows into the lumbar lymphatic trunks and cisterna chyli at the level of the second lumbar vertebra. From here, all the lymph is carried by the thoracic duct through the thorax with no intervening nodes to empty into the junction of the left subclavian and internal jugular veins.

Tumour cells that penetrate or bypass the pelvic and para-aortic nodes are rapidly disseminated via the great veins at the root of the neck.

Lymphatic drainage from the genital tract

The lymph vessel from individual parts of the genital tract drain into this system of pelvic lymph nodes in the following manner:

The vulva and perineum medial to the labiocrural skin folds contain superficial lymphatics which pass upwards towards the mons pubis, then curve laterally to the superficial and inguinal nodes. Drainage from these is through the fossa ovalis into the deep femoral nodes. The largest of these, lying in the upper part of the femoral canal, is known as the node of Cloquet.

The lymphatics of the lower third of the vagina follow the vulval drainage to the superficial lymph nodes, whereas those from the upper two thirds pass upwards to join the lymphatic vessels of the cervix.

The lymphatics of the cervix pass either laterally in the base of the broad ligament or posteriorly along the uterosacral ligaments to reach the side wall of the pelvis. Most of the vessels drain to the internal iliac obturator and external iliac nodes, but vessels also pass directly to the common iliac and lower para-aortic nodes. Radical surgery for carcinoma of the cervix should include removal of all these node groups on both sides of the pelvis.

Most of the lymphatic vessels of the body of the uterus join those of the cervix and therefore reach similar groups of nodes. A few vessels at the fundus follow the ovarian channels and there is an inconsistent pathway along the round ligament to the inguinal nodes.

The ovary and Fallopian tube have a plexus of vessels which drain along the infundibulopelvic fold to the para-aortic nodes on both sides of the midline. On the left, these are found around the left renal pedicle, while on the right there may only be one node intervening before the lymph flows into the thoracic duct thus accounting for the rapid early spread of metastatic carcinoma to distant sites such as the lungs.

The lymphatic drainage of the bladder and upper urethra is to the iliac nodes, while those of the lower part of the urethra follow those of the vulva.

Lymphatics from the lower anal canal drain to the superficial inguinal nodes and the remainder of the rectal drainage follows pararectal channels accompanying the blood vessels to both the internal iliac nodes (middle rectal artery) and the para-aortic nodes and the origin of the inferior mesenteric artery.

Nerves of the pelvis

Nerve supply of the vulva and perineum

The pudendal nerve arises form the second, third and fourth sacral nerves. As it passes along the outer wall of the ischiorectal fossa, it gives off an inferior rectal branch and divides into the perineal nerve and dorsal nerve of the clitoris (Figure 2.7). The perineal nerve gives the sensory supply to the vulva and also innervates the anterior part of the external anal canal and levator ani and the superficial perineal muscles. The dorsal nerve of the clitoris is sensory. Sensory fibres from the mons and labia also pass in the ilioinguinal and genitofemoral nerves to the first lumbar root. The posterior femoral cutaneous nerve carries sensation from the perineum to the small sciatic nerve and thus to the first second and third sacral nerves. The main nerve supply of the levator ani muscles comes from the third and fourth sacral nerves.

Nerve supply of the pelvic viscera

The innervation of the pelvic viscera is complex and not well understood. All pelvic viscera receive dual innervation, i.e both sympathetic and parasympathetic. Nerve fibres of the preaortic plexus

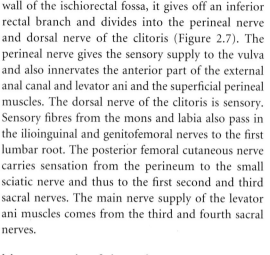
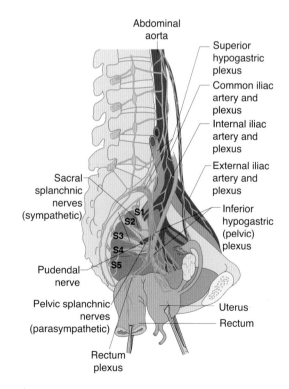

Figure 2.7   Nerve supply to the pelvis.

of the sympathetic nervous system are continuous with those of the superior hypogastric plexus which lies in front of the last lumber vertebra and is wrongly called the 'presacral nerve'. Below this, the superior hypogastric plexus divides and on each side its fibres are continuous with fibres passing beside the rectum to join the uterovaginal plexus (inferior hypogastric plexus or plexus of Frankenhauser). This plexus lies in the loose cellular tissue posterolateral to the cervix, below the uterosacral folds of peritoneum. Parasympathetic fibres from the second, third and fourth sacral nerves join the uterovaginal plexus. Fibres from (or to) the bladder, uterus, vagina and rectum join the plexus. The uterovaginal plexus contains a few ganglion cells, so it is likely that a few motor cells also have their relay stations there and then pass onward with the blood vessels onto the viscera.

The ovary is not innervated by the nerves already described, but from the ovarian plexus which surrounds the ovarian vessels and joins the preaortic plexus high up.

Key Points

- The paramesonephric duct which later forms the Mullerian system is the precursor of female genital development.

- The lower end of the Mullerian ducts fuse in the midline to form the uterus and upper vagina.

- Most of the upper vagina is of Mullerian origin, while the lower vagina forms from the sinovaginal bulbs.

- The primitive gonad is first evident at 5 weeks of embryonic life and forms on the medial aspect of the mesonephric ridge.

- The maximum number of primordial follicles is reached at 20 weeks gestation. These reduce by atresia throughout childhood and adult life.

- The size and ratio of the cervix to uterus changes with age and parity.

- Vaginal pH is normally acidic and has a protective role for decreasing the growth of pathogenic organisms.

- An adult uterus consists of three layers: the peritoneum, myometrium and endometrium.

- The cervix is narrower than the body of the uterus and is approximately 2.5 cm in length. The ureter runs about 1 cm lateral to the cervix.

- The epithelium of the cervix in its lower third is stratified squamous epithelium and the junction between this and the columnar epithelium is where most cervical carcinomas arise.

- The ovary is the only intraperitoneal structure not covered by peritoneum.

- The main supports to the pelvic floor are the connective tissue and levator ani muscles. The main supports of the uterus are the uterosacral ligaments which are condensations of connective tissue.

- The ovarian arteries arise directly from the aorta, while the right ovarian vein drains into the vena cava and the left into the left renal vein.

- The major nerve supply of the pelvis comes from the pudendal nerves which arise from the second, third and fourth sacral nerves.

CHAPTER 3

NORMAL AND ABNORMAL SEXUAL DEVELOPMENT AND PUBERTY

OVERVIEW

Sexual differentiation and development are highly complex processes which start at conception. A thorough understanding of these mechanisms is fundamental in understanding how the normal fetus develops. It is also key to understanding the complex group of conditions known as 'disorders of sex development' (DSD).

Sexual differentiation

Differentiation of the fertilized embryo into a male or female fetus is controlled by the sex chromosomes. All normal fetuses have an undifferentiated gonad which has the potential to become either a testis or an ovary. In addition, all fetuses have both Mullerian and Wolffian ducts and the potential to develop male or female internal and external genitalia. The chromosomal complement of the zygote determines whether the indifferent gonad becomes a testis or an ovary. The first step in this pathway is dependent on the SRY gene (sex determining region of the Y chromosome). This gene, helped by other testes-determining genes, causes the gonad to begin development into a testis. In the past, ovarian development was considered a 'default' development due solely to the absence of SRY, however, recently ovarian-determining genes have also been found.

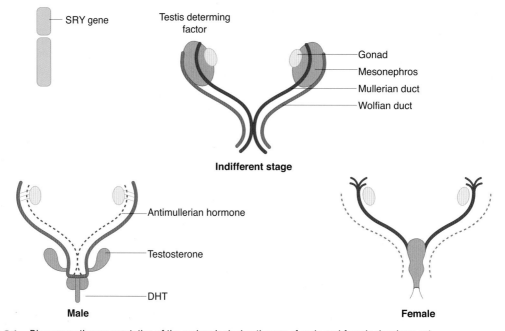

Figure 3.1 Diagrammatic representation of the embryological pathways of male and female development.

As the gonad develops into a testis, it differentiates into two cell types. The Sertoli cells produce anti-Mullerian hormone (AMH) and the Leydig cells produce testosterone. Anti-Mullerian hormone suppresses development of the Mullerian ducts. Testosterone stimulates the Wolffian ducts to develop into the vas deferens, epididymis and seminal vesicles. In addition, in the external genital skin, testosterone is converted by an enzyme called 5-alpha-reductase into dihydrotestosterone (DHT). This acts to virilize the external genitalia. The genital tubercle becomes the penis and the labioscrotal folds fuse to form the scrotum. The urogenital folds fuse along the ventral surface of the penis and include the urethra so that it opens at the tip of the penis.

Where the gonad becomes an ovary, the absence of AMH allows the Mullerian structures to develop. The proximal two thirds of the vagina develops from the paired Mullerian ducts which grow in a caudal and medial direction and fuse in the midline. These ducts form bilateral Fallopian tubes, and midline fusion of these structures produces the uterus, cervix and upper vagina. The rudimentary distal vagina fuses with the posterior urethra at week 7 to form the urogenital sinus. The vagina then develops from a combination of the Mullerian tubercles and the urogenital sinus. Cells proliferate from the upper portion of the urogenital sinus to form structures called the 'sinovaginal bulbs'. These fuse to form the vaginal plate which extends from the Mullerian ducts to the urogenital sinus. This plate begins to canalize, starting at the hymen and proceeds upwards to the cervix. A diagrammatic representation of the basic pathways is given in Figure 3.1.

The external genitalia do not virilize and, in the absence of testosterone, the genital tubercle becomes the clitoris and the labioscrotal swellings form the labia. The lower part of the vagina is formed from the urogenital folds.

Disorders of sex development

Disorders of sex development are conditions where the sequence of events described above does not happen. The clinical consequences of this depend upon where within the sequence the variation occurs. These may be diagnosed at birth with ambiguous or abnormal genitalia, but may also be seen at puberty

in girls who present with primary amenorrhoea or increasing virilization.

There has been a recent change in the terminology used to refer to these conditions. Older terms, such as 'hermaphrodite' and 'intersex', are confusing to both the clinician and patients, and in addition can be hurtful. The new terminology is summarized in Table 3.1.

Table 3.1   Summary of New Terminology for Disorders of Sex Development (DSD).

Previous	Proposed
Intersex	Disorders of Sex Development
Male pseudohermaphrodite Undervirilization of xy male Undermasculinization of xy male	46, XY DSD
Female pseudohermaphrodite Overvirilization of an XX female Masculinization of an XX female	46 XX DSD
True hermaphrodite	Ovotesticular DSD

Chromosomal abnormalities

Turner syndrome

If an embryo loses one of its sex chromosomes, then the total complement of chromosomes is 45. This is usually incompatible with life, except in the case of Turner syndrome which results from a complete or partial absence on one X chromosome (45XO). Turner syndrome is the most common chromosomal anomaly in females, occurring in 1 in 2500 live female births. Although there can be variation among affected women, most have typical clinical features including short stature, webbing of the neck and a wide carrying angle. Associated medical conditions include coarctation of the aorta, inflammatory bowel disease, sensorineural and conduction deafness, renal anomalies and endocrine dysfunction, such as autoimmune thyroid disease.

In this condition, the ovary does not complete its normal development and only the stroma is present at birth. The gonads are called 'streak gonads' and do not function to produce oestrogen or oocytes. Diagnosis is usually made at birth or in early childhood from the clinical appearance of the baby or due to short stature during childhood. However, in about 10 per cent of women, the diagnosis is not made until adolescence with delayed puberty. The ovaries do not produce oestrogen, so the normal physical changes of puberty cannot happen. In childhood, treatment is focused on growth, but in adolescence it focuses on induction of puberty. Pregnancy is possible, but ovum donation is usually required. Psychological input and support is important.

XY gonadal dysgenesis

In this situation, the gonads do not develop into a testis, despite the presence of an XY karyotype. In about 10 per cent of cases, this is due to an absent SRY gene, but in most cases the cause is unknown. In complete gonadal dysgenesis (Swyer syndrome), the gonad remains as a streak gonad and does not produce any hormones. In the absence of AMH, the Mullerian structures do not regress and the uterus, vaginal and Fallopian tubes develop normally. The absence of testosterone mean the fetus does not virilize. The baby is phenotypically female, although has an XY chromosome. The gonads do not function and presentation is usually at adolescence with failure to go into spontaneous puberty. The dysgenetic gonad has a high malignancy risk and should be removed when the diagnosis is made. This is usually performed laparoscopically. Puberty must be induced with oestrogen and pregnancies have been reported with a donor oocyte. Full disclosure of the diagnosis including the XY karytoype is essential, although can be devastating and psychological input is crucial.

Mixed gonadal dysgenesis is a more complex condition. The karyotype may be 46 XX, but mosaicism, e.g. XX/XY, is present in up to 20 per cent. In this situation, both functioning ovarian and testicular tissue can be present and if so this condition is known as ovotesticular DSD. The anatomical findings vary depending on the function of the gonads. For example, if the testes is functional, then the baby will virilize and have ambiguous or normal male genitalia. The Mullerian structures are usually absent on the side of the functioning testes, but a unicorcuate uterus may be present if there is an ovary or streak gonad.

46XY DSD

Complete androgen insensitivity syndrome (CAIS) occurs in individuals where virilization of the external genitalia does not occur due to a partial or complete inability of the androgen receptor to respond to androgen stimulation. In the fetus with CAIS, testes form normally due to the action of the SRY gene. At the appropriate time, these testes secrete AMH leading to the regression of the Mullerian ducts. Hence, CAIS women do not have a uterus. Testosterone is also produced at the appropriate time, however, due to the inability of the androgen receptor to respond, the external genitalia do not virilize and instead undergo female development. A female fetus is born with normal female external genitalia, an absent uterus and testes found at some point in their line of descent through the abdomen from the pelvis to the inguinal canal. During puberty, breast development will be normal, however, the effects of androgens are not seen, so pubic and axillary hair growth will be minimal. Presentation is usually at puberty with primary amenorrhoea, although if the testes are in the inguinal canal they can cause a hernia in a younger girl. Once the diagnosis is made, initially management is psychological with full disclosure of the XY karyotype and the information that the patient will be infertile. Gonadectomy is recommended because of the small long-term risk of testicular malignancy, although this can be deferred until after puberty. Once the gonads are removed, long-term hormone replacement therapy will be required. The vagina is usually shortened and treatment will be required to create a vagina suitable for penetrative intercourse. Vaginal dilation is the most effective method of improving vaginal length and entails the insertion of vaginal moulds of gradually increasing length and width for at least 30 minutes a day (Figure 3.2). Surgical vaginal reconstruction operations are reserved for those women that have failed a dilation treatment programme.

In cases of partial androgen insensitivity, the androgen receptor can respond to some extent with limited virilization. The child is usually diagnosed at birth with ambiguous genitalia.

5-Alpha-reductase deficiency

In this condition, the fetus has an XY karytype and a normal functioning testes which produce both testosterone and AMH. However, the fetus is unable

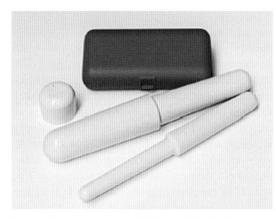

Figure 3.2 Femmax vaginal dilators. Dilation is the first line of treatment for women with a shortened or absent vagina, such as in MRKH syndrome.

to convert testosterone to dihydrotestosterone in the peripheral tissues and so cannot virilize normally. Presentation is usually with ambiguous genitalia at birth, but can also be with increasing virilization at puberty of a female child due to the large increase in circulating testosterone with the onset of puberty. In the Western world, the child is usually assigned to a female sex of rearing, but there have been descriptions of a few communities where transition from a female to male gender at puberty is accepted.

Congenital adrenal hyperplasia

This condition leads to virilization of a female fetus. It is due to an enzyme deficiency in the corticosteroid production pathway in the adrenal gland with over 90 per cent being a deficiency in 21-hydroxylase, which converts progesterone to deoxycorticosterone, and 17-hydroxyprogesterone (17-OHP) to deoxycortisol. The reduced levels of cortisol being produced drive the negative feedback loop, resulting in hyperplasia of the adrenal glands and increased levels of progesterone production. This leads to an excess of androgen precursors and then to elevated testosterone production. Raised androgen levels in a female fetus will lead to virilization of the eternal genitalia. The clitoris is enlarged and the labia are fused and scrotal in appearance. The upper vagina joins the urethra and opens as one common channel onto the perineum. In addition, two thirds of children with 21-OH CAH will have a 'salt-losing' variety, which also affects the

ability to produce aldosterone. This represents a life-threatening situation, and those children who are salt-losing often become dangerously unwell within a few days of birth. Affected individuals require life-long steroid replacement, such as hydrocortisone – along with fludrocortisone for salt losers. Once the infant is well and stabilized on their steroid regime, surgical treatment of the genitalia is considered. Traditionally, all female infants with CAH underwent feminizing genital surgery within the first year of life. This management is now controversial as adult patients with CAH are very dissatisfied with the outcome of their surgery and argue that surgery should have been deferred until they were old enough to have a choice. Surgery certainly leaves scarring and may reduce sexual sensitivity, but the alternative of leaving the genitalia virilized throughout childhood can be difficult for parents to consider. At present, cases are managed individually by a multidisciplinary team involving surgeons, endocrinologists and psychologists.

Mullerian anomalies

These are common, occurring in up to 6 per cent of the female population, and may be asymptomatic. The aetiology is unknown, although associated renal anomalies are present in up to 30 per cent.

Mullerian obstruction

Failure of complete canalization of the Mullerian structures can lead to menstrual obstruction. The obstruction most commonly occurs at the junction of the lower third of the vagina at the level of the hymen, although more proximal obstruction can occur. Presentation with an imperforate hymen is usually with increasing abdominal pain in a girl in early adolescence. The retained menstrual blood stretches the vagina causing a haematocolpus. This can cause a large pelvic mass and in addition can usually be seen as a bulging membrane at the vaginal entrance. Treatment is simple with a surgical incision of the hymen and drainage of the retained blood.

Mullerian duplication

Duplication of the Mullerian system can occur resulting in a wide range of anomalies. It may be a complete duplication of the uterus, cervix and vagina,

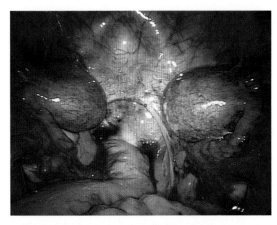

Figure 3.3 Laparoscopic view of bilateral rudimentary uterine horns. This patient presented with primary amenorrhoea and had a short blind-ending vagina.

but may be simply a midline uterine septum in otherwise normal internal genitalia. Second uterine horns may also occur and can be rudimentary or functional (Figure 3.3).

Mullerian agenesis

In approximately 1 in 5000 to 1 in 40 000 girls, the Mullerian system does not develop resulting in an absent or rudimentary uterus and upper vagina. This condition is known as Rokitansky syndrome or Mayer–Rokitansky–Kuster–Hauser (MRKH) syndrome. The ovaries function normally and so the most common presentation is with primary amenorrhoea in the presence of otherwise normal pubertal development. The aetiology of this condition is not known although possible culprits include environmental, genetic, hormonal or receptor factors. On examination, the vagina will be blind ending and is likely to be shortened in length. An ultrasound scan will confirm the presence of ovaries, but no functioning uterus will be present. Treatment options focus on psychological support and on the creation of a vagina comfortable for penetrative intercourse, as described above for CAIS. There is currently no treatment available to transplant a uterus in humans, although there is extensive ongoing research being undertaken in this area. Women with MRKH syndrome may have their own genetic children, using ovum retrieval and assisted conception techniques, and a surrogate mother.

Normal puberty

Puberty is the process of reproductive and sexual development and maturation which changes a child into an adult. During childhood, the hypothalamic–pituitary–ovarian axis is suppressed and levels of GnRH, FSH and LH are very low. However, from the age of eight to nine years, GnRH is secreted in pulsations of increasing amplitude and frequency. These are initially sleep-related, but as puberty progresses, these extend throughout the day. This stimulates secretion of FSH and LH by the pituitary glands which in turn triggers follicular growth and steroidogenesis in the ovary. The oestrogen produced by the ovary then initiates the physical changes of puberty. The exact mechanism determining the onset of puberty is still unknown, but it is influenced by many factors including race, heredity, body weight and exercise. Leptin plays a permissive role in the onset of puberty.

The physical changes occurring in puberty are:

- breast development (thelarche);
- pubic and axillary hair growth (adrenarche);
- growth spurt;
- onset of menstruation (menarche).

The first physical signs of puberty are breast budding and this occurs two or three years before menarche. The appearance of pubic hair is dependent on the secretion of adrenal androgens and is usually after thelarche. In addition to increasing levels of adrenal and gonadal hormones, growth hormone secretion also increases leading to a pubertal growth spurt. The mean age of menarche is 12.8 years and it may take over three years before the menstrual cycle establishes a regular pattern. Initial cycles are usually anovulatory and can be unpredictable and irregular. Pubertal development was described by Tanner and the stages of breast and pubic hair development are often referred to as Tanner stages 1 to 5 (Figure 3.4).

Precocious puberty

This is defined as the onset of puberty before the age of eight in a girl or nine in a boy. It is classified as either central or peripheral. Central precocious puberty is gonadotrophin-dependent. The aetiology is often unknown, although up to 25 per cent are due to central nervous system malformation or brain tumours. Peripheral precocious puberty is always

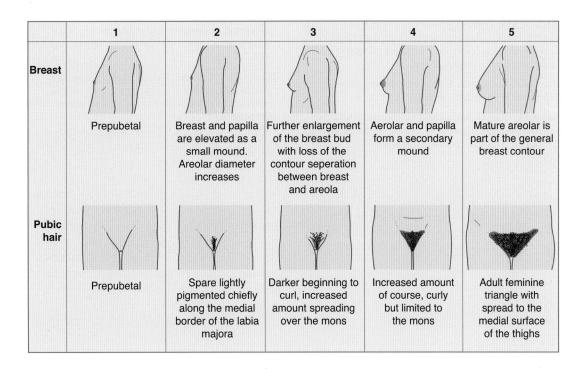

	1	2	3	4	5
Breast	Prepubetal	Breast and papilla are elevated as a small mound. Areolar diameter increases	Further enlargement of the breast bud with loss of the contour seperation between breast and areola	Aerolar and papilla form a secondary mound	Mature areolar is part of the general breast contour
Pubic hair	Prepubetal	Spare lightly pigmented chiefly along the medial border of the labia majora	Darker beginning to curl, increased amount spreading over the mons	Increased amount of course, curly but limited to the mons	Adult feminine triangle with spread to the medial surface of the thighs

Figure 3.4   Tanner staging.

pathological and can be caused by oestrogen secretion, such as exogenous ingestion or a hormone-producing tumour.

Delayed puberty

This occurs when there are no signs of secondary sexual characteristics by the age of 14 years. It is due to either a central defect – hypogonadotrophic hypogonadism or to a failure of gonadal function – hypergonadotrophic hypogonadism.

Hypogonadotrophic hypogonadism

This may be constitutional, but other causes must be excluded. These include anorexia nervosa, excessive exercise and chronic illness, such as diabetes or renal failure. Rarer causes include a pituitary tumour and Kalmans syndrome.

Hypergonadotrphic hypogonadism

In this situation, the gonad does not function despite a high FSH. Both Turner syndrome and XX gonadal dysgenesis will cause this. Premature ovarian failure can occur at any age and may be idiopathic, but can also be part of an autoimmune disorder or following chemo- or radiotherapy for childhood cancer.

Key Points

- Sex differentiation is determined by the presence of the SRY region of the Y chromosome, although other testes- and ovarian-determining genes have a role.
- Older terms, such as hermaphrodite and intersex, have been replaced by the term 'disorder of sex development' (DSD).
- Presentation of a DSD is most commonly at birth with ambiguous genitalia or at puberty with virilization or primary amenorrhoea.
- A multidisciplinary team is essential for the management of patients with a DSD.
- Turner syndrome is the most common chromosomal anomaly in girls and has typical clinical features.
- Puberty is a well-defined progression of physical changes from the child to adult and any abnormalities in this progression warrant investigation.

Additional reading

Androgen Insensitivity Syndrome Support Group (AISSG). Available from: www.aissg.org.uk.

Goswami D, Conway GS. Premature ovarian failure. *Hormone Research* 2007; **68**: 196–202.

Hughes IA, Houk C, Ahmed SF, Lee PA. Consensus statement on management of intersex disorders. *Archives of Disease in Childhood* 2006; **91**: 554–63.

Michala L, Goswami D, Creighton SM, Conway GS. Swyer syndrome: presentation and outcomes. *BJOG: An International Journal of Obstetrics and Gynaecology* 2008; **115**: 737–41.

Ogilvie CM, Crouch NS, Rumsby G *et al*. Congenital adrenal hyperplasia in adults: a review of medical, surgical and psychological issues. *Clinical Endocrinology* 2006; **64**: 2–11.

CHAPTER 4

THE NORMAL MENSTRUAL CYCLE

OVERVIEW

It is important to have an understanding of the physiology of the normal menstrual cycle to understand the causes of any abnormalities, and also to tackle problems, such as infertility and the prevention of unwanted pregnancy. This chapter aims to describe the mechanisms involved in the normal menstrual cycle, with emphasis on the clinical relevance of each phase.

Introduction

The external manifestation of a normal menstrual cycle is the presence of regular vaginal bleeding. This occurs as a result of the shedding of the endometrial lining following failure of fertilization of the oocyte or failure of implantation. The cycle depends on changes occurring within the ovaries and fluctuation in ovarian hormone levels, that are themselves controlled by the pituitary and hypothalamus, the hypothalamo–pituitary–ovarian axis (HPO).

Hypothalamus

The hypothalamus in the forebrain secretes the peptide hormone gonadotrophin-releasing hormone (GnRH), which in turn controls pituitary hormone secretion. GnRH must be released in a pulsatile fashion to stimulate pituitary secretion of luteinizing hormone (LH) and follicle stimulating hormone (FSH). If GnRH is given in a constant high dose, it desensitizes the GnRH receptor and reduces LH and FSH release.

Drugs that are GnRH agonists (e.g. buserelin and goserelin) can be used as treatments for endometriosis and other gynaecological problems. Although they mimic the GnRH hormone, when administered continuously, they will downregulate the pituitary and consequently decrease LH and FSH secretion. This has effects on ovarian function such that oestrogen and progesterone levels also fall, and most women using these analogues become amenorrhoeic. These preparations are used as treatments for endometriosis and to shrink fibroids prior to surgery.

Pituitary gland

GnRH stimulation of the basophil cells in the anterior pituitary gland causes synthesis and release of the gonadotrophic hormones, FSH and LH. This process is modulated by the ovarian sex steroid hormones oestrogen and progesterone (see Figure 4.1). Low levels of oestrogen have an inhibitory effect on LH production (negative feedback), whereas high levels of oestrogen will increase LH production (positive feedback). The mechanism of action for the positive feedback effect of oestrogen involves an increase in GnRH receptor concentrations, while the mechanism of the negative feedback effect is uncertain.

The high levels of circulating oestrogen in the late follicular phase of the ovary act via the positive feedback mechanism to generate a periovulatory LH surge from the pituitary.

The clinical relevance of these mechanisms is seen in the use of the combined oral contraceptive pill, which artificially creates a constant serum oestrogen level in the negative feedback range, inducing a correspondingly low level of gonadotrophin hormone release.

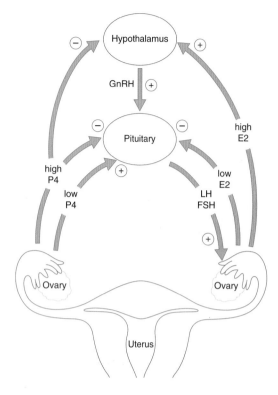

Figure 4.1   Hypothalamo–pituitary–ovarian axis.

Ovary

Ovaries with developing oocytes are present in the female fetus from an early stage of development. By the end of the second trimester *in utero*, the number of oocytes has reached a maximum and they arrest at the first prophase step in meiotic division. No new oocytes are formed during the female lifetime. With the onset of menarche, the primordial follicles containing oocytes will activate and grow in a cyclical fashion, causing ovulation and subsequent menstruation in the event of non-fertilization.

In the course of a normal menstrual cycle, the ovary will go through three phases:

1 Follicular phase

2 Ovulation

3 Luteal phase.

Follicular phase

The initial stages of follicular development are independent of hormone stimulation. However, follicular development will fail at the preantral stage and follicular atresia will ensue if pituitary hormones LH and FSH are absent.

FSH levels rise in the first days of the menstrual cycle, when oestrogen, progesterone and inhibin levels are low. This stimulates a cohort of small antral follicles on the ovaries to grow.

Within the follicles, there are two cell types which are involved in the processing of steroids, including oestrogen and progesterone. These are the theca and the granulosa cells, which respond to LH and FSH stimulation, respectively. LH stimulates production of androgens from cholesterol within theca cells. These androgens are converted into oestrogens by the process of aromatization in granulosa cells, under the influence of FSH. The roles of FSH and LH in follicular development are demonstrated by studies on women undergoing ovulation induction in whom endogenous gonadotrophin production has been suppressed. If pure FSH alone is used for ovulation induction, an ovulatory follicle can be produced, but oestrogen production is markedly reduced. Both FSH and LH are required to generate a normal cycle with adequate amounts of oestrogen.

As the follicles grow and oestrogen secretion increases, there is negative feedback on the pituitary

Unlike oestrogen, low levels of progesterone have a positive feedback effect on pituitary LH and FSH secretion (as seen immediately prior to ovulation) and contribute to the FSH surge. High levels of progesterone, as seen in the luteal phase, inhibit pituitary LH and FSH production. Positive feedback effects of progesterone occur via increasing sensitivity to GnRH in the pituitary. Negative feedback effects are generated through both decreased GnRH production from the hypothalamus and decreased sensitivity to GnRH in the pituitary. It is known that progesterone can only have these effects on gonadotropic hormone release after priming by oestrogen (Figure 4.2).

In addition to these well-known hormones, there are other hormones which are involved in pituitary gonadotrophin secretion. Inhibin and activin are peptide hormones produced by granulosa cells in the ovaries, with opposing effects on gonadotrophin production. Inhibin inhibits pituitary FSH secretion, whereas activin stimulates it.

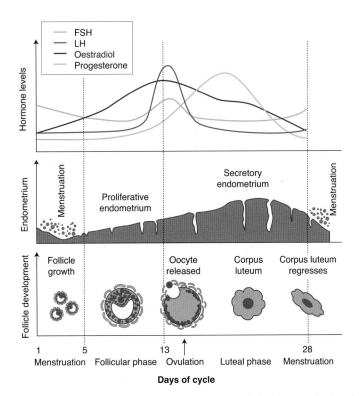

Figure 4.2   Changes in hormone levels, endometrium and follicle development during the menstrual cycle.

to decrease FSH secretion. This assists in the selection of one follicle to continue in its development towards ovulation – the dominant follicle. In the ovary, the follicle which has the most efficient aromatase activity and highest concentration of FSH-induced LH receptors will be the most likely to survive as FSH levels drop, while smaller follicles will undergo atresia. The dominant follicle will go on producing oestrogen and also inhibin, which enhances androgen synthesis under LH control.

Ovarian stimulation beyond the control of the normal hypothalamo–pituitary–ovarian axis will not progress in the manner described above, as it is dependent on appropriate gonadotrophic hormone response from the pituitary controlling the follicular development. Administration of exogenous gonadotrophins is likely to stimulate growth of multiple follicles which continue to develop and are released at ovulation (and can lead to multiple gestations at a rate of around 30 per cent).

This situation is used to advantage in patients requiring *in vitro* fertilization (IVF), as many oocytes can be harvested from ovaries which have been

stimulated as described above. They can then undergo fertilization *in vitro*, and surviving embryos can be chosen for transfer back to the uterus.

There are other autocrine and paracrine mediators playing a role in the follicular phase of the menstrual cycle. These include inhibin and activin. Inhibin is produced in men in the testicles to inhibit pituitary FSH production. In women, it is secreted by the granulosa cells within the ovaries. It participates in feedback to the pituitary to downregulate FSH release, and also appears to enhance ongoing androgen synthesis. Activin is structurally similar to inhibin, but has an opposite action. It is produced in granulosa cells and in the pituitary, and acts to increase FSH binding on the follicles.

Insulin-like growth factors (IGF-I, IGF-II) act as paracrine regulators. Circulating levels do not change during the menstrual cycle, but follicular fluid levels increase towards ovulation, with the highest level found in the dominant follicle. The actions of IGF-I and -II are modified by their binding proteins: insulin-like growth factor binding proteins (IGFBPs). In the follicular phase, IGF-I is produced by theca cells under the action of LH. IGF-I receptors are present on both theca and granulosa cells. Within the theca, IGF-I augments LH-induced steroidogenesis. In granulosa cells, IGF-I augments the stimulatory effects of FSH on mitosis, aromatase activity and inhibin production. In the preovulatory follicle, IGF-I enhances LH-induced progesterone production from granulosa cells. Following ovulation, IGF-II is produced from luteinized granulosa cells, and acts in an autocrine manner to augment LH-induced proliferation of granulosa cells.

Kisspeptins are proteins which have more recently been found to play a role in regulation of the HPO axis, via the mediation of the metabolic hormone leptin's effect on the hypothalamus. Leptin is thought to be key in the relationship between energy production, weight and reproductive health. Mutations in the kisspeptin receptor, gpr-54, are associated with delayed or absent puberty, probably due to a reduction in leptin-linked triggers for gonadotrophin release.

Ovulation

By the end of the follicular phase, which lasts an average of 14 days, the dominant follicle has grown to approximately 20 mm in diameter. As the follicle matures, FSH induces LH receptors on the granulosa cells to compensate for lower FSH levels and prepare for the signal for ovulation. Production of oestrogen increases until they reach the necessary threshold to exert a positive feedback effort on the hypothalamus and pituitary to cause the LH surge. This occurs over 24–36 hours, during which time the LH-induced luteinization of granulosa cells in the dominant follicle causes progesterone to be produced, adding further to the positive feedback for LH secretion and causing a small periovulatory rise in FSH. Androgens, synthesized in the theca cells, also rise around the time of ovulation and this is thought to have an important role in stimulating libido, ensuring that sexual activity is likely to occur at the time of greatest fertility.

The LH surge is one of the best predictors of imminent ovulation, and this is the hormone detected in urine by most over-the-counter 'ovulation predictor' tests.

The LH surge has another function in stimulating the resumption of meiosis in the oocyte just prior to its release. The physical ovulation of the oocyte occurs after breakdown of the follicular wall occurs under the influence of LH, FSH and progesterone-controlled proteolytic enzymes, such as plasminogen

activators and prostaglandins. There appears to be an inflammatory-type response within the follicle wall which may assist in extrusion of the oocyte by stimulating smooth muscle activity.

Studies have shown that inhibition of prostaglandin production may result in failure of ovulation. Thus, women wishing to become pregnant should be advised to avoid taking prostaglandin synthetase inhibitors, such as aspirin and ibuprofen, which may inhibit oocyte release.

Luteal phase

After the release of the oocyte, the remaining granulosa and theca cells on the ovary form the corpus luteum. The granulosa cells have a vacuolated appearance with accumulated yellow pigment, hence the name corpus luteum ('yellow body'). The corpus luteum undergoes extensive vascularization in order to supply granulosa cells with a rich blood supply for continued steroidogenesis. This is aided by local production of vascular endothelial growth factor (VEGF).

Ongoing pituitary LH secretion and granulosa cell activity ensures a supply of progesterone which stabilizes the endometrium in preparation for pregnancy. Progesterone levels are at their highest in the cycle during the luteal phase. This also has the effect of suppressing FSH and LH secretion to a level that will not produce further follicular growth in the ovary during that cycle.

The luteal phase lasts 14 days in most women, without great variation. In the absence of beta human chorionic gonadotrophin (βHCG) being produced from an implanting embryo, the corpus luteum will regress in a process known as luteolysis. The mature corpus luteum is less sensitive to LH, produces less progesterone, and will gradually disappear from the ovary. The withdrawal of progesterone has the effect on the uterus of causing shedding of the endometrium and thus menstruation. Reduction in levels of progesterone, oestrogen and inhibin feeding back to the pituitary cause increased secretion of gonadotrophic hormones, particularly FSH. New preantral follicles begin to be stimulated and the cycle begins anew.

Endometrium

The hormone changes effected by the HPO axis during the menstrual cycle will occur whether the uterus is present or not. However, the specific secondary changes in the uterine endometrium give the most obvious external sign of regular cycles.

Menstruation

The endometrium is under the influence of sex steroids that circulate in females of reproductive age. Sequential exposure to oestrogen and progesterone will result in cellular proliferation and differentiation, in preparation for the implantation of an embryo in the event of pregnancy, followed by regular bleeding in response to progesterone withdrawal if the corpus luteum regresses. During the ovarian follicular phase, the endometrium undergoes proliferation (the 'proliferative phase'); during the ovarian luteal phase, it has its 'secretory phase'. Decidualization, the formation of a specialized glandular endometrium, is an irreversible process and apoptosis occurs if there is no embryo implantation. Menstruation (day 1) is the shedding of the 'dead' endometrium and ceases as the endometrium regenerates (which normally happens by day 5–6 of the cycle).

The endometrium is composed of two layers, the uppermost of which is shed during menstruation. A fall in circulating levels of oestrogen and progesterone approximately 14 days after ovulation leads to loss of tissue fluid, vasoconstriction of spiral arterioles and distal ischaemia. This results in tissue breakdown, and loss of the upper layer along with bleeding from fragments of the remaining arterioles is seen as menstrual bleeding. Enhanced fibrinolysis reduces clotting.

The effects of oestrogen and progesterone on the endometrium can be reproduced artificially, for example in patients taking the combined oral contraceptive pill or hormone replacement therapy who experience a withdrawal bleed during their pill-free week each month.

Vaginal bleeding will cease after 5–10 days as arterioles vasoconstrict and the endometrium begins to regenerate. Haemostasis in the uterine endometrium is different from haemostasis elsewhere in the body as it does not involve the processes of clot formation and fibrosis.

In rare cases, the tissue breakdown and vasoconstriction does not occur correctly and the endometrium may develop scarring which goes on to inhibit its function. This is known as 'Asherman's syndrome'.

The endocrine influences in menstruation are clear. However, the paracrine mediators less so. Prostaglandin $F_2\alpha$, endothelin-1 and platelet activating factor (PAF) are vasoconstrictors which are produced within the endometrium and are thought likely to be involved in vessel constriction, both initiating and controlling menstruation. They may be balanced by the effect of vasodilator agents, such as prostaglandin E_2, prostacyclin (PGI) and nitric oxide (NO), which are also produced by the endometrium. Recent research has shown that progesterone withdrawal increases endometrial prostaglandin (PG) synthesis and decreases PG metabolism. The COX-2 enzyme and chemokines are involved in PG synthesis and this is likely to be the target of non-steroidal anti-inflammatory agents used for the treatment of heavy and painful periods.

Endometrial repair involves both glandular and stromal regeneration and angiogenesis to reconstitute the endometrial vasculature. VEGF and fibroblast growth factor (FGF) are found within the endometrium and both are powerful angiogenic agents. Epidermal growth factor (EGF) appears to be responsible for mediation of oestrogen-induced glandular and stromal regeneration. Other growth factors, such as transforming growth factors (TGFs) and IGFs, and the interleukins may also be important.

Greater understanding of mediators of menstruation is important in the search for medications to control heavy and painful periods. Mefenamic acid is a PG synthetase inhibitor which is widely used as a treatment for heavy menstrual bleeding. It is believed to act by increasing the ratio of the vasoconstrictor $PGF2\alpha$ to the vasodilator PGE_2. Mefenamic acid reduces menstrual loss by a mean value of 20–25 per cent in women with very heavy bleeding, and furthermore more effective agents are still being sought.

The proliferative phase

Menstruation will normally cease after 5–7 days, once endometrial repair is complete. After this time, the endometrium enters the proliferative phase, when glandular and stromal growth occur. The epithelium lining the endometrial glands changes from a single layer of columnar cells to a pseudostratified epithelium with frequent mitoses. The stroma is infiltrated by cells derived from the bone marrow (see Figure 4.3). Endometrial thickness increases rapidly, from 0.5 mm at menstruation to 3.5–5 mm at the end of the proliferative phase.

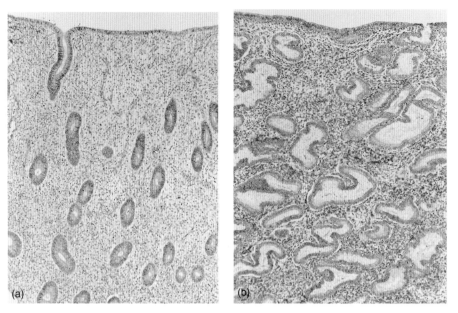

Figure 4.3   Tissue sections of normal endometrium during proliferative and secretory phases of the menstrual cycle.

The secretory phase

After ovulation (generally around day 14), there is a period of endometrial glandular secretory activity. Following the progesterone surge, the oestrogen-induced cellular proliferation is inhibited and the endometrial thickness does not increase any further. However, the endometrial glands will become more tortuous, spiral arteries will grow, and fluid is secreted into glandular cells and into the uterine lumen. Later in the secretory phase, progesterone induces the formation of a temporary layer, known as the decidua, in the endometrial stroma. Histologically, this is seen as occurring around blood vessels. Stromal cells show increased mitotic activity, nuclear enlargement and generation of a basement membrane (see Figure 4.3).

Recent research into infertility has identified apical membrane projections of the endometrial epithelial cells known as pinopodes, which appear after day 21–22 and appear to be a progesterone-dependent stage in making the endometrium receptive for embryo implantation (see Figure 4.4).

Immediately prior to menstruation, three distinct layers of endometrium can be seen. The basalis is the lower 25 per cent of the endometrium, which will

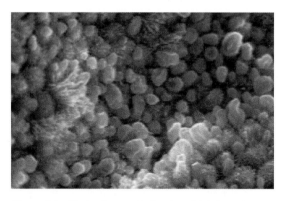

Figure 4.4   Photomicrograph of endometrial pinopodes from the implantation window.

remain throughout menstruation and shows few changes during the menstrual cycle. The mid-portion is the stratum spongiosum with oedematous stroma and exhausted glands. The superficial portion (upper 25 per cent) is the stratum compactum with prominent decidualized stromal cells. On the withdrawal of both oestrogen and progesterone, the decidua will collapse, with vasoconstriction and relaxation of spiral arteries and shedding of the outer layers of the endometrium.

New developments

Measurement of ovarian reserve

Female reproductive potential is directly proportionate to the remaining number of oocytes in the ovaries. This number decreases from birth onwards, and the rate of loss accelerates after the age of 37 in an average healthy woman, or at an earlier age following long-term gonadotrophin deficit or exposure to toxins, e.g. chemotherapy. It is desirable to be able to quantify the residual ovarian capacity of women of older age or after undergoing treatment in order to give prognostic information and management advice to patients, and also to compare different forms of treatment. Research using ultrasound markers has looked at measurements of ovarian volume, mean ovarian diameter and antral follicle count to calculate ovarian reserve. Biochemical markers include FSH, oestradiol, inhibin B, anti-Mullerian hormone (AMH). AMH is produced in the granulosa cells of ovarian follicles and does not change in response to gonadotrophins during the menstrual cycle. As a result, it can be measured and compared from any point in the cycle.

Harvesting ovarian tissue

Harvesting and cryopreservation of ovarian tissue is an emerging technique in reproductive biology. At present, its use is experimental and offered to nulliparous women or young females undergoing gonadotrophic therapy, for example to treat cancer. The theory is that strips of ovarian cortex can be removed at laparoscopy or laparotomy and preserved by freezing, in the hope that future technology will allow them to be thawed and used to generate oocytes for IVF treatment.

Key Points

Menstruation

- Menstruation occurs in response to changing levels of oestrogen and progesterone.
- Endometrial shedding is initiated largely by arteriolar vasoconstriction and involves the upper 75 per cent of the endometrial lining.
- Menstruation stops due to vasoconstriction and endometrial repair.
- Fibrinolysis inhibits scar tissue formation.

Proliferative phase

- Oestrogen induces growth of glands and stroma.

Secretory phase

- Progesterone induces glandular secretory activity.
- Pinopodes form in the mid-secretory phase and make the endometrium receptive for implantation.
- Decidualization occurs in the late secretory phase.

OVERVIEW

Disorders of the menstrual cycle are one of the most common reasons for women to attend their general practitioner and, subsequently, a gynaecologist. Although rarely life threatening, menstrual disorders can cause major social, psychological and occupational upset.

Heavy menstrual bleeding

There has been some confusion over the various terminologies used for abnormalities of menstrual blood loss. Heavy menstrual bleeding (HMB) is now the preferred description as it is simple and easily translatable into other languages. It replaces the older term 'menorrhagia' (Table 5.1).

HMB is defined as a blood loss of greater than 80 mL per period. In reality, methods to quantify menstrual blood loss are both inaccurate (poor correlation with haemoglobin level) and impractical and so a clinical diagnosis based on the patient's own perception of blood loss is preferred.

The presentation of HMB is common because women are having fewer children and consequently more menstrual cycles. Indeed, each year in the UK, 5 per cent of women between the ages of 30 and 49 consult their general practitioner with this complaint, with a substantial number being referred on to secondary care.

Table 5.1 Symptoms which can be associated with HMB and related pathologies

Associated symptoms	Suggestive of:

Irregular bleeding
  Intermenstrual bleeding
  Postcoital bleeding
	Endometrial or cervical polyp

Excessive bruising/bleeding from other sites History of postpartum haemorrhage (PPH) Excessive postoperative bleeding Excessive bleeding with dental extractions Family history of bleeding problems	Coagulation disorder (Coagulation disorders will be present in 20% of those presenting with 'unexplained' heavy menstrual bleeding.)
Unusual vaginal discharge	Pelvic inflammatory disease
Urinary symptoms	Pressure from fibroids
Weight change, skin changes, fatigue	Thyroid disease

Aetiology

- Fibroids (Figure 5.1)
- Endometrial polyps (Figure 5.2)
- Coagulation disorders, e.g. von Willebrand's disease
- Pelvic inflammatory disease (PID)
- Thyroid disease
- Drug therapy (e.g. warfarin)
- Intrauterine contraceptive devices (IUCDs)
- Endometrial/cervical carcinoma.

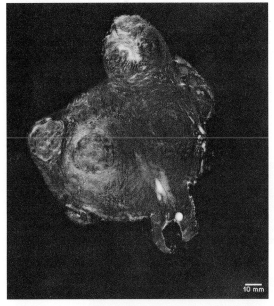

Figure 5.1 7T image of fibroid uterus (image courtesy of Dr KI Munro).

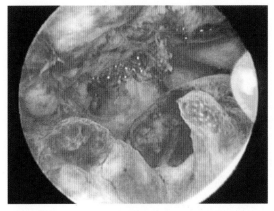

Figure 5.2 Hysteroscopic view of an endometrial polyp (image courtesy of Dr AW Horne).

Despite appropriate investigations, often no pathology can be identified. Bleeding of endometrial origin (BEO) is the diagnosis of exclusion. This replaces the older 'dysfunctional uterine bleeding' (DUB). Disordered endometrial prostaglandin production has been implicated in the aetiology of BEO, as have abnormalities of endometrial vascular development.

History and examination

Patients will have different ideas as to what constitutes a 'heavy period' (see Table 5.1). Useful questions include:

- How often does soaked sanitary wear need to be changed?
- Is there presence of clots?
- Is the bleeding so heavy (flooding) that it spills over your towel/tampon and on to your pants, clothes or bedding?
- Have you had to take any time off work due to this bleeding? Do you ever find you are confined to your house when the bleeding is at its worst?

After examining the patient for signs of anaemia, it is important to perform an abdominal and pelvic examination in all women complaining of HMB. This enables any pelvic masses to be palpated, the cervix to be visualized for polyps/carcinoma, swabs to be taken if pelvic infection is suspected or a cervical smear to be taken if one is due.

Investigations

Full blood count

A full blood count (FBC) should be carried out in all women with HMB to ascertain the need for iron therapy (and in certain cases, blood transfusion).

Coagulation screen

Referral for a haematological opinion should be considered in women with a history consistent with a coagulation disorder (see Table 5.1).

Pelvic ultrasound scan

A pelvic ultrasound scan (USS) should be performed:

- when a pelvic mass is palpated on examination (suggestive of fibroids);
- when symptoms suggest an endometrial polyp, e.g. irregular or intermenstrual bleeding;
- when drug therapy for HMB is unsuccessful.

High vaginal and endocervical swabs

High vaginal and endocervical swabs should be taken:

- when unusual vaginal discharge is reported or observed on examination;
- where there are risk factors for PID.

Endometrial biopsy

Biopsy should be performed:

- in those aged >45 years;
- if irregular or intermenstrual bleeding;
- drug therapy has failed.

A Pipelle™ endometrial biopsy can be performed in the outpatient setting. It is performed as follows:

- a speculum examination is carried out and the cervix is completely visualized;
- a vulsellum instrument may be required to grasp the cervix and provide gentle traction, thereby straightening the endocervical canal;
- the Pipelle sampler (Figure 5.3) is carefully inserted through the cervical os until it reaches the fundus of the uterus. The length of the uterus is noted;
- the inner part of the Pipelle is withdrawn to create a vacuum and the device is gently moved in and out to obtain a sample of endometrial tissue;
- the Pipelle is removed and the tissue is expelled into a histopathology container of formalin.

An outpatient hysteroscopy (Figure 5.4) with endometrial biopsy may be indicated if:

- Pipelle biopsy attempt fails;
- Pipelle biopsy sample is insufficient for histopathology assessment;
- there is an abnormality on USS, e.g. suggested endometrial polyp or submucosal fibroid;
- patient is known to poorly tolerate speculum examinations (more comfortable vaginoscopic approach can be used).

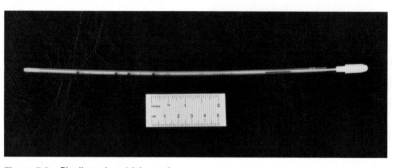

Figure 5.3   Pipelle endometrial sampler.

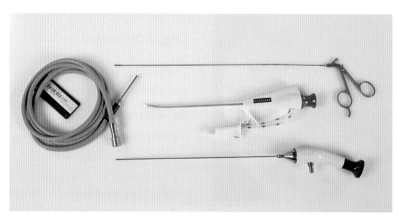

Figure 5.4   Hysteroscope.

If the patient fails to tolerate an outpatient procedure or the cervix needs to be dilated to enter the cavity, then a hysteroscopy and endometrial biopsy under general anaesthetic may be required.

Thyroid function tests

This should only be carried out when the history is suggestive of a thyroid disorder.

Management

For some women, the demonstration that their blood loss is in fact 'normal' may be sufficient to reassure them and make further treatment unnecessary. For others, there are a number of different treatments for HMB. The effectiveness of medical treatments is often temporary, while surgical treatments are mostly incompatible with desired fertility.

When selecting appropriate management for the patient, it is important to consider and discuss:

- the patient's preference of treatment;
- risks/benefits of each option;
- contraceptive requirements:
  - family complete?
  - current contraception?
- past medical history:
  - any contraindications to medical therapies for HMB?
  - suitability for an anaesthetic. Previous surgical history?

Medical treatments

The British National Formulary (BNF) should be consulted for a detailed list of contraindications, cautions and side effects for each drug before prescription to patients.

Mefenamic acid and other non-steroidal anti-inflammatory drugs

Mefenamic acid and other non-steroidal anti-inflammatory drugs (NSAIDs) are associated with a reduction in mean menstrual blood loss of 20–25 per cent. This may be sufficient in some women to restore menstrual blood loss either to normal or to a level which is compatible with a reasonable quality of life.

- Benefits: Effective analgesia, hence often the first-line treatment of choice where dysmenorrhoea coexists.
- Disadvantages: Contraindicated with a history of duodenal ulcer or severe asthma.
- Recommended dose: 500 mg p.o. tds to be taken when menstruation is particularly heavy or painful.

Although not a BNF contraindication, there are some recent concerns that long-term usage of NSAIDs may cause reversible difficulties in conceiving (see Chapter 4, The normal menstrual cycle).

Tranexamic acid

This is associated with a mean reduction in menstrual blood loss (MBL) of about 50 per cent. Theoretical concerns have been raised that tranexamic acid may be associated with an increased risk of venous thrombosis, but this has not been borne out by the studies that have investigated it to date.

- Benefits: Only requires to be taken on days when the bleeding is particularly heavy. It is compatible with ongoing attempts at conception.
- Recommended dose: 1 g p.o. qds to be taken when menstruating heavily.

Combined oral contraceptive pill

- Benefits: Doubles up as a very effective contraceptive when taken properly.
- Disadvantages: (1) It is contraindicated for patients who have risk factors for thromboembolism. (2) It is unsuitable for patients over 35 years old who smoke. (3) It is unsuitable if there is a personal or family history of breast cancer. (4) It is unsuitable for patients who are grossly overweight.

Norethisterone

This cyclical progestogen is effective taken in a cyclical pattern from day 6 to day 26 of the menstrual cycle.

- Benefits: It is a safe and effective oral preparation, which can regulate bleeding pattern.
- Disadvantages: It is not a contraceptive and can cause break-through bleeding.

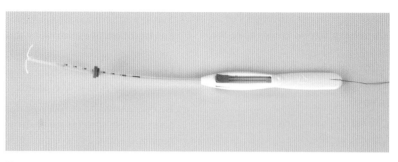

Figure 5.5   The levonorgestrel intrauterine system (LNG-IUS, Mirena).

- Recommended dose: 5–10 mg tds on days 6–26 of the menstrual cycle.

Levonogestrel intrauterine system

The levonogestrel intrauterine system (LNG-IUS, Mirena™) (Figure 5.5) has revolutionized the treatment of HMB as it provides a highly effective alternative to surgical treatment, with few side effects. Indeed, the Royal College of Obstetricians and Gynaecologists (RCOG) has suggested that the LNG-IUS should be considered in the majority of women as an alternative to surgical treatment. Mean reductions in MBL of around 95 per cent by one year after LNG-IUS insertion have been demonstrated.

- Benefits:
  - It provides contraceptive cover comparable with sterilization.
  - Recent evidence proves it is effective for associated dysmenorrhoea.
  - Around 30 per cent of women are amenorrhoeic by one year after insertion.
- Disadvantages:
  - Irregular menses and break-through bleeding for the first three to nine months after insertion.

GnRH agonists

These drugs act on the pituitary to stop the production of oestrogen which results in amenorrhoea. These are only used in the short term due to the resulting hypo-oestrogenic state which predisposes to osteoporosis.

- Benefits:
  - They are effective for associated dysmenorrhoea.
- Disadvantages:
  - They can cause irregular bleeding.

- They can be associated with flushing and sweating.
- Only suitable for short-term usage (six months) unless combined with addback hormone replacement therapy (HRT).
- Dose:
  - Goserelin (Zoladex™) 3.6 mg monthly subcutaneous implant
  - Decapeptyl (Triptorelin™) 3 mg monthly or 11.25 mg three-monthly subcutaneous or intramuscular injection;
  - Buserelin (Suprecur™) 300 μg nasal spray tds.

Surgical treatments

Surgical treatment is normally restricted to women for whom medical treatments have failed. Women contemplating surgical treatment for HMB must be certain that their family is complete. While this caveat is obvious for women contemplating hysterectomy, in which the uterus will be removed, it also applies to women contemplating endometrial ablation. Therefore women wishing to preserve their fertility for future attempts at childbearing should be advised to use medical methods of treatment. The risks of a pregnancy after an ablation procedure theoretically include prematurity and morbidly adherent placenta.

Endometrial ablation

All endometrial destructive procedures employ the principle that ablation of the endometrial lining of the uterus to sufficient depth prevents regeneration of the endometrium. The mean reduction in blood loss associated with this procedure is estimated at around 90 per cent. The first-generation techniques, including transcervical resection of the endometrium with

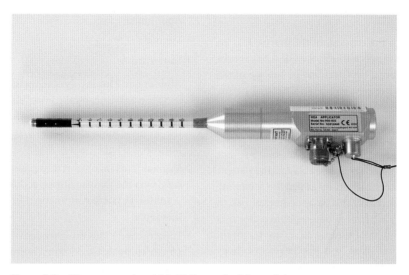

Figure 5.6   Microwave endometrial ablation probe (Microsulis).

electrical diathermy loop or rollerball ablation, have largely been replaced by newer second-generation techniques. These include:

- Impedence controlled endometrial ablation (Novasure™)
- Thermal uterine balloon therapy (Thermachoice™)
- Microwave ablation (Microsulis™) (Figure 5.6).

Success rates

As a general rule, of all women undergoing endometrial ablation with a second-generation technique, 40 per cent will become amenorrhoeic, 40 per cent will have markedly reduced menstrual loss and 20 per cent will have no difference in their bleeding. Some authorities have suggested that endometrial ablation is so successful that all women with HMB should be encouraged to consider it before opting for hysterectomy. While there are merits to this argument, some women, after informed discussion, will still prefer hysterectomy and they should therefore be considered for this procedure instead.

The procedure

- This takes place as an outpatient or day-case procedure either performed with local anaesthetic in the outpatient setting or under general anaesthetic in theatre.
- It is performed through the cervix.

- Hysteroscopy precedes the ablation and should be repeated following the procedure.
- The full thickness of the endometrium is ablated by controlled application of energy in the form of heat or microwave.
- The newer second-generation techniques offer a shorter learning curve for the operator, quicker treatment times and lower complication rates.

Pre-procedure

The patients must be appropriately counselled prior to their procedure. The following should be included in the discussion:

- a description of the endometrial ablation procedure;
- success rates of the procedure;
- risks of the procedure (uterine perforation, haemorrhage, fluid overload);
- recovery time;
- alternative treatment options to endometrial ablation;
- need for contraception.

Post-procedure

- Symptoms to expect: crampy pain for 24 hours and light bleeding or greyish vaginal discharge for up to a few weeks.
- Plan for contraception.

Hysterectomy

A hysterectomy is the removal of the uterus. It is an extremely common procedure in the UK – 20 per cent of women will have a hysterectomy by the age of 60. Interestingly, 40 per cent will have a normal uterus on histological examination. Subtotal hysterectomy (STAH) is removal of the uterus while the cervix remains. This is carried out when the patient states this as her preference or when adhesions prevent safe removal of the cervix. With a STAH the patient will still require cervical smears as per the screening programme as there will still be a theoretical risk of cervical cancer. A bilateral salpingo-oopherectomy is where both ovaries and Fallopian tubes are removed. In counselling the patient, it is important to convey that removal of the ovaries will result in an immediate post-menopausal state with varying degrees of systemic oestrogen withdrawal symptoms, including flushing, sweating and mood changes, in addition to an increased risk of osteoporosis. Hormone replacement therapy may need to be considered. Where the ovaries remain *in situ*, there is always a risk of future disease, including ovarian cysts or ovarian carcinoma. Therefore, a thorough personal and family history (ovarian and breast cancer) is essential. Removal of the uterus and ovaries without the woman's consent (or without her full understanding of the nature of the procedure) is a recurrent cause of litigation in gynaecology. It is essential, therefore, to obtain express consent for each part of the procedure before embarking on hysterectomy.

Pre-procedure

The patient must be appropriately counselled. The discussion should include:

- a description of the procedure;
- the removal or retaining of ovaries and cervix (see above);
- risks of the procedure (anaesthetic risk, haemorrhage, infection, bowel, bladder or ureteric damage, deep vein thrombosis, pulmonary embolus);
- recovery time (see below);
- alternative treatment options to hysterectomy.

Procedure

A hysterectomy may be achieved using three approaches:

1 Abdominal
2 Vaginal
3 Laparoscopic.

1 Abdominal: This involves an incision which is usually transverse, on the lower abdomen. A vertical midline incision is sometimes used if the uterus is markedly enlarged, for example, by fibroids.

2 Vaginal: This involves removal of the uterus and cervix via the vagina with no abdominal incisions. A subtotal hysterectomy cannot be performed via this route.

3 Laparoscopic: This category can be subdivided. Laparoscopy-assisted vaginal hysterectomy (LAVH) is where part of the hysterectomy is performed laparoscopically and part vaginally. Total laparoscopic hysterectomy (TLH) is where the whole procedure is performed laparoscopically. This 'keyhole' approach requires only small incisions on the abdomen.

Both the laparoscopic and vaginal approaches result in a quicker return to normal activities and a shorter hospital stay. Where the uterus is not enlarged, these techniques should be used in preference to the abdominal approach if appropriate. However, the laparoscopic approach involves a longer operating time and requires a certain level of surgical expertise. The vaginal approach has the highest risk of pelvic haematoma with an incidence of around 30 per cent.

Post-procedure

- Regular observations.
- Regular analgesia.
- A urinary catheter inserted preoperatively will remain in the bladder for 24 hours.
- The patient will remain in hospital for 3–5 days.
- Wound sutures/staples will be removed 7–10 days postoperatively,
- The recovery time is 6–12 weeks.
- Thrombo-embolic prophylaxis.

Dysmenorrhoea

Dysmenorrhoea is defined as painful menstruation. It is experienced by 45–95 per cent of women of reproductive age. There may not be identifiable pelvic pathology. There is some evidence to support the assertion that dysmenorrhoea improves after childbirth, and it also appears to decline with increasing age.

Aetiology

Aetiology includes:

- endometriosis and adenomyosis;
- pelvic inflammatory disease;
- cervical stenosis and haematometra (rarely).

Endometriosis

Endometriosis, most prevalent in patients of reproductive age, is the presence of endometrial tissue outside the uterine cavity including the ovary, the pelvic walls, the pouch of Douglas, the uterosacral ligaments and the bowel. These patches of ectopic tissue are under hormonal influence and hence symptoms are exacerbated at the time of menstruation. Laparoscopy is the 'gold standard' diagnostic tool. Treatment options include the combined pill (best taken continuously), the Mirena IUS or a surgical approach with laser, diathermy or excision of endometriotic tissue. Complications of endometriosis include the formation of adhesions, 'chocolate' ovarian cysts (endometriomas) and infertility. Adenomyosis is the presence of ectopic endometrial tissue within the myometrium. It is associated with previous procedures which may break the barrier between the endometrium and the myometrium, e.g. Caesarean section or suction termination of pregnancy.

History and examination

Patients will have different ideas as to what constitutes a painful period. To ascertain the severity of the pain, the following questions may be useful:

- Do you need to take painkillers for this pain? Which tablets help?
- Have you needed to take any time off work/school due to the pain?

An abdominal and pelvic examination should be performed. Certain signs associated with endometriosis include a pelvic mass (if an endometrioma is present), a fixed uterus (if adhesions are present) and endometriotic nodules (palpable in the pouch of Douglas or on the uterosacral ligaments).

Investigation

High vaginal and endocervical swabs

These should be carried out to exclude pelvic infection, in particular *Chlamydia trachomatis* and *Neisseria gonorrhoea*.

Pelvic ultrasound scan

Pelvic ultrasound scan may be useful to detect endometriomas or appearances suggestive of adenomyosis (enlarged uterus with heterogeneous texture).

Diagnostic laparoscopy

Diagnostic laparoscopy if performed:

- when the history is suggestive of endometriosis;
- when swabs and USS are normal, yet symptoms persist;
- when the patient wants a definite diagnosis or wants reassurance that their pelvis is normal.

    Discussion about laparoscopy should include:

- the risks of the procedure, including anaesthetic complications, damage to blood vessels/bladder/bowel and infection;
- the fact that this investigation may show no obvious causes for their symptoms.

If features in the history suggest cervical stenosis, ultrasound and hysteroscopy can be used to investigate further. However, this condition is an infrequent cause of dysmenorrhoea, and this investigation should not be routine.

Management

Non-steroidal anti-inflammatory drugs

NSAIDs are effective in a large proportion of women. Some examples are naproxen, ibuprofen and mefenamic acid.

Oral contraceptives

These are widely used but, surprisingly, a recent review of randomized controlled trials provides little evidence supporting this treatment as being effective.

LNG-IUS

There is recent evidence that this is beneficial for dysmenorrhoea and indeed can be an effective treatment for underlying causes, such as endometriosis and adenomyosis.

Lifestyle changes

There is some evidence to suggest that a low fat, vegetarian diet may improve dysmenorrhoea. There are suggestions that exercise may improve symptoms by improving blood flow to the pelvis.

GnRH analogues

This is not a first-line treatment nor an option for prolonged management due to the resulting hypo-oestrogenic state. These are best used to manage symptoms if awaiting hysterectomy or as a form of assessment as to the benefits of hysterectomy. If the pain does not settle with the GnRH analogue, it is unlikely to be resolved by removing the ovaries at hysterectomy.

Heat

Although this may seem a rather old-fashioned method for helping dysmenorrhoea, there is strong evidence to prove its benefit. It appears to be as effective as NSAIDs.

Dyspareunia

Dyspareunia is defined as pain during sexual intercourse. This can be superficial or deep, the latter sometimes associated with pathology such as endometriosis or pelvic inflammatory disease. On many occasions, despite appropriate investigations, no cause can be found and psychological support should be offered.

Amenorrhoea/oligomenorrhoea

Amenorrhoea is defined as the absence of menstruation.

- Primary amenorrhoea is when girls fail to menstruate by 16 years of age.
- Secondary amenorrhoea is absence of menstruation for more than six months in a normal female of reproductive age that is not due to pregnancy, lactation or the menopause.

Anatomical disorders

- Genital tract abnormalities;
- Asherman's syndrome;
- Mullerian agenesis;
- transverse vaginal septum;
- imperforate hymen.

Asherman's syndrome is the presence of intrauterine adhesions which prevent menstruation, the most common cause being over-vigorous uterine curettage. Mullerian agenesis is a congenital malformation where the Mullerian ducts fail to develop resulting in an absent uterus and variable malformations of the vagina.

Ovarian disorders

Ovarian disorders include the following:

- anovulation (polycystic ovarian syndrome, see below);
- premature ovarian failure (POF).

POF is defined as cessation of periods before 40 years of age. It is usually unexplained, but may be due to chemotherapy, radiotherapy, autoimmune disease or chromosomal disorders (e.g. Turner's 45XO/46XX).

Pituitary disorders

- Adenomas of which prolactinoma is most common.
- Pituitary necrosis, e.g. Sheehan's syndrome (due to prolonged hypotension following major obstetric haemorrhage).

Hypothalamic disorders

- Excessive exercise, weight loss and stress can switch off hypothalamic stimulation of the pituitary
- Hypothalamic lesions (craniopharyngioma, glioma) can compress hypothalamic tissue or block dopamine
- Head injuries
- Kallman's syndrome (X-linked recessive condition resulting in deficiency in GnRH causing underdeveloped genitalia)
- Systemic disorders including sarcoidosis, tuberculosis resulting in an infiltrative process in the hypothalamo-hypophyseal region
- Drugs: progestogens, HRT or dopamine antagonists.

Findings from the history should guide the examination (Table 5.2). A general inspection of the patient should be carried out to assess body mass index (BMI), secondary sexual characteristics (hair growth, breast development) and signs of endocrine abnormalities (hirsutism, acne, abdominal striae, moon-face, skin changes). If the history is suggestive of a pituitary lesion, an assessment of visual fields is indicated. External genitalia and a vaginal examination should be performed to detect structural outflow abnormalities or demonstrate atrophic changes consistent with hypo-oestrogenism.

Investigation of amenorrhoea/ oligomenorrhoea

Findings from the history and examination should guide the choice and order of investigations. A pregnancy test should be carried out if the patient is sexually active. Blood can be taken for LH, FSH and testosterone; raised LH or raised testosterone could be suggestive of polycystic ovarian syndrome (PCOS); raised FSH may be suggestive of POF. A raised prolactin level may indicate a prolactinoma. Thyroid function should be checked if clinically indicated. An USS can be useful in detecting the classical appearances of polycystic ovaries (see Figure 5.8) and magnetic resonance imaging (MRI) should be carried out if symptoms are consistent with a pituitary adenoma. Hysteroscopy is not routine, but is a suitable investigation where Asherman's or cervical stenosis is suspected. Karyotyping is diagnostic of Turner's. The management of amenorrhoea/oligomenorrhoea is outlined in Table 5.3.

Polycystic ovarian syndrome

PCOS is a syndrome of ovarian dysfunction along with the cardinal features of hyperandrogenism and polycystic ovary morphology (Figure 5.7). Its clinical manifestations include menstrual irregularities, signs of androgen excess (e.g. hirsutism) and obesity. Elevated serum LH levels and insulin resistance and are also common features. PCOS is associated with an increased risk of type 2 diabetes and cardiovascular

Table 5.2   History and examination of patient with amenorrhoea/oligomenorrhoea

Information required	Relevant factors	Possible diagnoses
Developmental history including menarche	Delayed/incomplete	Congenital malformation or chromosomal abnormality
Menstrual history	Oligomenorrhoea	PCOS
	Secondary amenorrhoea	POF
Reproductive history	Infertility	PCOS
		Congenital malformation
Cyclical symptoms	Cyclical pain without menstruation	Congenital malformation
		Imperforate hymen
Hair growth	Hirsutism	PCOS
Weight	Dramatic weight loss	Hypothalamic malfunction
	Difficulty losing weight	PCOS
Lifestyle	Exercise, stress	Hypothalamic malfunction
Past medical history	Systemic diseases, e.g. sarcoidosis	Hypothalamic malfunction
Past surgical history	Evacuation of uterus	Asherman's
Drug history	Dopamine agonists, HRT	Hypothalamic malfunction
Headache		Pituitary adenoma
Galactorrhoea		Prolactinoma
Visual disturbance		Pituitary adenoma

Table 5.3 Management of amenorrhoea/oligomenorrhoea

Cause of amenorrhoea/oligomenorrhoea	Management
Low BMI	Dietary advice and support
Hypothalamic lesions, e.g. glioma	Surgery
Hyperprolactinaemia/prolactinoma	Dopamine agonist (e.g. cabergoline or bromocriptine) or surgery if medication fails
POF	HRT or COCP
PCOS	See below
Asherman's	Adhesiolysis and IUD insertion at time of hysteroscopy (to prevent recurrence of adhesions)
Cervical stenosis	Hysteroscopy and cervical dilatation

events. It affects around 5–10 per cent of women of reproductive age. The prevalence of polycystic ovaries seen on ultrasound is much higher at around 25 per cent (Figure 5.8).

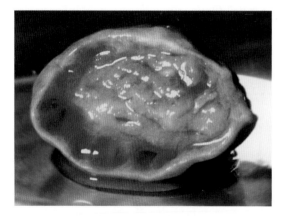

Figure 5.7 Gross appearance of polycystic ovary.

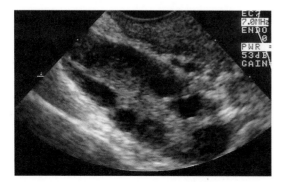

Figure 5.8 Ultrasound picture of polycystic ovary.

Aetiology

The aetiology of PCOS is not completely clear, but there is often a family history. It seems likely that a gene is important in its development.

Clinical features

The clinical features of PCOS are as follows:

- oligomenorrhoea/amenorrhoea in up to 75 per cent of patients, predominantly related to chronic anovulation;
- hirsutism;
- subfertility in up to 75 per cent of women;
- obesity in at least 40 per cent of patients;
- recurrent miscarriage in around 50–60 per cent of women;
- acanthosis nigricans (areas of increased velvety skin pigmentation occur in the axillae and other flexures);
- may be asymptomatic.

Diagnosis

Patients must have two out of the three features below:

- amenorrhoea/oligomenorrhoea;
- clinical or biochemical hyperandrogenism;
- polycystic ovaries on ultrasound.

The ultrasound criteria for the diagnosis of a polycystic ovary are eight or more subcapsular follicular cysts <10 mm in diameter and increased ovarian stroma.

While these findings support a diagnosis of PCOS, they are not by themselves sufficient to identify the syndrome.

Management

Management of PCOS involves the following:

- COCP: This should regulate menstruation.
- Cyclical oral progesterone: This too can be used to regulate menstruation.
- Metformin: This is beneficial in a subset of patients with PCOS, those with hyperinsulinaemia and cardiovascular risk factors. It is less effective than clomiphene for ovulation induction and it does not improve pregnancy outcome. It should be discontinued when pregnancy is detected.
- Clomiphene: This can be used to induce ovulation where subfertility is a factor.
- Lifestyle advice: Dietary modification and exercise is appropriate in these patients as they are at an increased risk of developing diabetes and cardiovascular disease later in life.
- Weight reduction.

Hirsutism

- Eflornithine cream (Vaniqua™) applied topically;
- Cyproterone acetate (Dianette™, anti-androgen contraceptive pill);
- Metformin: improves parameters of insulin resistance, hyperandrogenemia, anovulation and acne in PCOS;
- GnRH analogues with low-dose HRT: this regime should be reserved for women intolerant of other therapies;
- Surgical treatments, e.g. laser or electrolysis.

Post-menopausal bleeding

Post-menopausal bleeding (PMB) is defined as vaginal bleeding after the menopause. In women who are not taking HRT, any bleeding is abnormal. In women on combined cyclical HRT, bleeding in the progesterone-free period is normal. Unscheduled bleeding refers to bleeding at other times: this is abnormal and should always be investigated.

Aetiology

- atrophic vaginitis;
- endometrial polyps;
- endometrial hyperplasia;
- endometrial carcinoma;
- cervical carcinoma.

The majority of women with PMB will be found to have atrophic vaginitis, whereby the vaginal epithelium thins and breaks down in response to low oestrogen levels. This is a benign condition, which is relatively easily treated with topical oestrogens. However, 10 per cent of patients with PMB will have endometrial cancer, therefore all patients with PMB must have this diagnosis excluded promptly. The risk of endometrial cancer progressively increases with age.

History and examination

Some useful questions include:

- When was your last period? (i.e. confirm menopausal)
- Was the bleeding post-coital? (i.e. think cervical polyp/cervical malignancy)
- When was your last smear done? Have they always been normal? (i.e. think cervical malignancy).

Examination should include an abdominal and vaginal examination to detect any pelvic masses and a speculum to visualize the vaginal tissues for atrophy and the cervix for polyps or potential carcinoma. A smear should be taken if due.

Investigations

An ultrasound scan should be carried out in all women to assess endometrial thickness. If, at ultrasound, the endometrial thickness is 3 mm or less (or 5 mm or less for women on HRT) patients can be reassured that the likelihood of endometrial carcinoma is extremely low and no further investigation is required. For those with an endometrial thickness greater than 3 mm (5 mm for those on HRT), further endometrial assessment is warranted in the form of an endometrial biopsy.

The exception to this rule is women on tamoxifen as ultrasound will not assist with a diagnosis.

Table 5.4   Management of PMB

Diagnosis	Management
Atrophic vagnitis	Topical oestrogen cream, oestrogen pessaries or Estring™ oestrogen ring pessary
Cervival polyp	Remove via speculum examination using polyp forceps
Endometrial polyp	Remove under direct visualization at hysteroscopy
Simple hyperplasia	Progestogens: oral preparation or LNG-IUS (Mirena)
Complex hyperplasia	Progestogens: oral preparation or LNG-IUS (Mirena)
Atypical hyperplasia	Total abdominal hysterectomy as significant risk of progression to malignancy
Endometrial cancer	Total abdominal hysterectomy + BSO + washings ± adjuvant therapy

Most women on tamoxifen will have a thickened, irregular and cystic endometrium. Immediate direct visualization of the cavity by hysteroscopy and an endometrial biopsy is the investigation of choice for such women. Management of PMB is discussed in Table 5.4.

Endometrial cancer is most prevalent in the post-menopausal age group. It typically presents with PMB. Risk factors include nulliparity, obesity, early menarche, late menopause and tamoxifen exposure. Diagnosis is by endometrial biopsy. Endometrial cancer treatment should begin with staging which involves total abdominal hysterectomy with washings, bilateral salpingo-oophorectomy and lymph node evaluation. The need for postoperative adjuvant radiotherapy is determined by recurrence risk. Patients with disease confined to the endometrium with little or no invasion into uterine muscle uterus often require only surgery. Where the cancer has deeply invaded into the uterine muscle or spread outside the uterus, adjuvant therapy in the form of radio- or chemotherapy is indicated. The prognosis is good when the disease is detected early.

Premenstrual syndrome

Premenstrual syndrome (PMS) is the occurrence of cyclical somatic, psychological and emotional symptoms that occur in the luteal (premenstrual) phase of the menstrual cycle and resolve by the time menstruation ceases.

Premenstrual symptoms occur in almost all women of reproductive age. In 3–60 per cent, symptoms are severe, causing disruption to everyday life, in particular interpersonal relationships.

Aetiology

The precise aetiology of PMS is unknown, but cyclical ovarian activity and the effects of oestradiol and progesterone on certain neurotransmitters, including serotonin, appear to play a role.

History and examination

The patient is likely to complain of some or all of the following:

- bloating;
- cyclical weight gain;
- mastalgia;
- abdominal cramps;
- fatigue;
- headache;
- depression;
- irritability.

The cyclical nature of PMS is the cornerstone of the diagnosis. A symptom chart, to be filled in by the patient prospectively, may help.

Management

The management of premenstrual syndrome is depicted in Figure 5.9.

Simple therapies

Simple therapies include:

- stress reduction;
- alcohol and caffeine limitation;
- exercise.

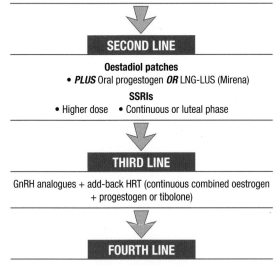

FIRST LINE

Lifestyle modifications
• Stress reduction • Exercise • Dietary changes

COCP
Ideally continuous

SSRIs
• Low dose • Continuous or luteal phase

Cognitive behavioural therapy

SECOND LINE

Oestadiol patches
• *PLUS* Oral progestogen *OR* LNG-LUS (Mirena)

SSRIs
• Higher dose • Continuous or luteal phase

THIRD LINE

GnRH analogues + add-back HRT (continuous combined oestrogen + progestogen or tibolone)

FOURTH LINE

Total abdominal hysterectomy and bilateral oophorectomy. + HRT (including testosterone)

Figure 5.9 Suggested management of premenstrual syndrome (adapted with permission from Panay N. Management of premenstrual syndrome. *Journal of Family Planning and Reproductive Health Care* 2009; **35**: 187–93).

Medical treatments

Combined oral contraceptive pill

The most effective preparation appears to be Yasmin™, which contains an anti-mineralocorticoid and an anti-androgenic progestogen. The most effective regime appears to be bicycling or tricycling pill packets (i.e. taking two or three packets in a row without a scheduled break).

Transdermal oestrogen

This has been shown to significantly reduce PMS symptoms.

GnRH analogues

GnRH analogues are a very effective treatment for PMS as ovarian activity is switched off. However, this

is generally a short-term treatment. If used for more than six months, HRT should be given to reduce the risk of osteoporosis.

Selective serotonin reuptake inhibitors

There is good evidence that this group of drugs significantly improve PMS.

Hysterectomy with bilateral salpingo-oopherectomy

This procedure obviously completely removes the ovarian cycle. It should only be performed if all other treatments have failed. It is essential for such patients to have a preoperative trial of GnRH analogue as a 'test' to ensure that switching off ovarian function (by removing the ovaries at hysterectomy) will indeed cure the problem.

Vitamins

Initial studies suggest that magnesium, calcium and isoflavones may be useful in treating PMS.

Alternative therapies

Initial results of St John's Wort are promising, particularly in improving mood. Although Evening

Key Points

- Heavy menstrual bleeding (HMB) is now the preferred terminology over menorrhagia.

- Twenty per cent of all women presenting with HMB will have an underlying coagulation disorder.

- Many women with HMB do not have any underlying pathology.

- The LNG-IUS (Mirena) is a highly effective form of medical management in the treatment of HMB and should be considered as an alternative to surgical procedures.

- Despite its wide use for dysmenorrhoea, there is no proven evidence that the COCP is effective for this problem.

- The second-generation endometrial ablation techniques offer an effective, safe and minimally invasive alternative to hysterectomy.

- There are a range of evidence-based modes of treatment for severe PMS and hysterectomy should only be used when all of these have failed.

- Unscheduled post-menopausal bleeding should always be investigated and endometrial carcinoma excluded.

CASE HISTORY

Miss B is a 22-year-old, para 0 + 0 who presents with a history of painful periods. They have always been painful since the menarche aged 13. The pains are getting worse. Her periods are regular with a 4–5/28-day cycle. She uses condoms for contraception and has recently been finding intercourse increasingly painful. She is slim and otherwise well. Her mother also had painful periods resulting in a hysterectomy in her 30s.

What is the most likely diagnosis?

Given the history of worsening dysmenorrhoea and dyspareunia, a likely diagnosis is endometriosis.

What else would you want to elicit from the history?

- Usage of analgesia?

- Any restrictions on daily activity?

- A sexual history should be taken to assess risk for pelvic inflammatory disease, which could be a differential diagnosis.

- Associated symptoms: HMB, intermenstrual/postcoital bleeding?

- Is the dyspareunia is superficial or deep?

What might you find on examination?

- Tenderness

- Palpable endometrial nodules

- Reduced mobility of uterus

- Adnexal mass (if endometriotic ovarian cyst present)

What investigations would help confirm the diagnosis?

- Endocervical and high vaginal swabs should be taken to exclude PID

- An ultrasound scan will probably be normal, but would exclude the presence of an endometrioma.

- A diagnostic laparoscopy should be considered.

What treatment options should be discussed with the patient?

- Analgesia in the form of NSAIDs

- COCP

- LNG-IUS (Mirena)

- GnRH agonists

- Surgical management at the time of laparoscopy with laser or diathermy.

primrose oil is commonly used, there is no evidence to support this treatment for PMS.

Cognitive-behavioural therapy

Cognitive-behavioural therapy (CBT) appears to be particularly effective when combined with selective serotonin reuptake inhibitors (SSRIs).

Additional reading

Amant F. Moerman P, Neven P *et al*. Endometrial cancer. *Lancet* 2005; **366**: 491–505.

Brown J, O'Brien PMS, Marjoribanks J, Wyatt K. Selective serotonin reuptake inhibitors for premenstrual syndrome (Review). *Cochrane Database of Systematic Reviews* 2009; (**2**): CD001396.

Munro MG, Lukes AS. Abnormal uterine bleeding and underlying haemostatic disorders: report of a consensus process. *Fertility and Sterility* 2005; **84**: 1335–7.

Nalaboff KM, Pellerito JS, Ben-Levi E. Imaging the endometrium: disease and normal variants. *Radiographics* 2001; **21**: 1409–24.

National Institute for Health and Clinical Excellence. Heavy menstrual bleeding. NICE Clinical Guideline CG44, 2007. Available from: www.nice.org.uk.

Nieboer TE, Johnson N, Lethaby A *et al*. Surgical approach to hysterectomy for benign gynaecological disease (review). *Cochrane Database of Systemic Reviews* 2009; (**3**): CD3677.

Panay N. Management of premenstrual syndrome. *Journal of Family Planning and Reproductive Health Care* 2009; **35**: 187–93.

Proctor M, Farquhar C. Diagnosis and management of dysmenorrhoea. *British Medical Journal* 2006; **332**: 1134–8.

Warner PE, Critchley HO, Lumsden MA. Referral for menstrual problems: cross-sectional survey of symptoms, reasons for referral, and management. *British Medical Journal* 2001; **323**: 24–8.

Warner PE, Critchley HO, Lumsden MA *et al*. Menorrhagia II: is the 80 ml blood loss criterion useful in management of complaint of menorrhagia? *American Journal of Obstetrics and Gynaecology* 2004; **192**: 2093.

Wong CL, Farquhar C, Roberts H, Proctor M. Oral contraceptive pill as treatment for primary dysmenorrhoea. *Cochrane Database of Systematic Reviews* 2009; (**4**): CD002120.

Woolcock JG, Critchley HO, Munro MG *et al*. Review of the confusion in current and historical terminology and definitions for disturbances of menstrual bleeding. *Fertility and Sterility* 2008; **90**: 2269–80.

CHAPTER 6

GENITAL INFECTIONS IN GYNAECOLOGY

OVERVIEW

Genital infections are one of the most common reasons for women of all age groups to present to a medical practitioner. Sexually transmitted infections form one subgroup of infections, however the more common infections are vulvovaginal candidiasis and bacterial vaginosis. Chlamydia and gonorrhoea affect the sexually active woman, with HIV being less common in the United Kingdom. These infections can be asymptomatic and can have serious consequences to a woman's fertility by causing tubal infection and damage. Appropriate diagnosis and treatment are fundamental not only to provide symptom relief, but also to prevent recurrences and long-term sequelae.

Introduction

It is important to differentiate normal physiological changes from true infections. Thus, a thorough history and examination with the back up of laboratory testing is fundamental before a diagnosis is made. However, the sensitivity of clinical diagnosis and testing in pelvic inflammatory disease (PID) can be low, so if there is a clinical suspicion of PID, empiric treatment is recommended. It is important to understand the implications of labelling someone with an infection, as it can have serious psychological and sexual implications in a relationship.

Anatomy and physiology

The vaginal epithelium is lined by stratified squamous epithelium during the reproductive age group under the influence of oestrogen. The pH is usually between 3.5 and 4.5 and lactobacilli (Figure 6.1a) are the most common organisms present in the vagina. Following the menopause, the influence of oestrogen is diminished making the vaginal epithelium atrophic with a more alkaline pH of 7.0, the lactobacillus population declines and the vagina is colonized by skin flora.

Physiological discharge occurs in response to hormonal levels during the menstrual cycle. It is usually white and changes to a more yellowish colour due to oxidation on contact with air. There is increased mucous production from the cervix at the time of ovulation followed by a thicker discharge/cervical plug under the influence of progesterone. The discharge mainly consists of mucous, desquamated epithelial cells, bacteria (lactobacillius) and fluid.

Ascending infection can occur from the vagina and cervix to the uterine cavity and to the Fallopian tubes through direct spread or via the lymphatics leading to severe pelvic inflammatory disease and pelvic peritonitis.

Infections can be broadly divided into lower and upper genital tract depending on the site and affection of the infective organism.

Lower genital tract infections

Vulvovaginal candidiasis

This is one of the most common genital infections and is caused by *Candida albicans* in around 80–92 per cent of cases. Other non-albican species like *C. tropicalis*, *C. glabrata*, *C. krusei* and *C. parapsilosis* can also cause similar symptoms, although sometimes more severe and recurrent. *C. albicans* is a diploid fungus and is a common commensal in the gut flora.

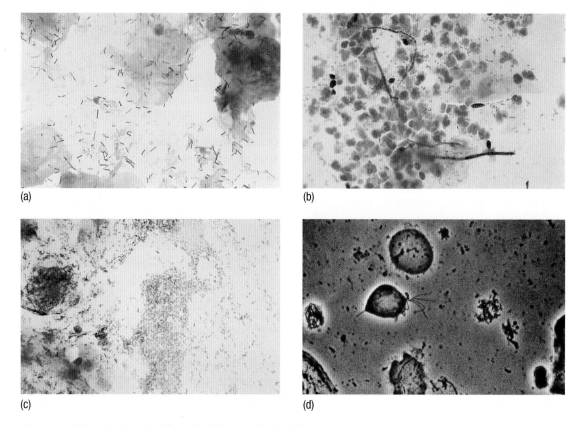

(a)

(b)

(c)

(d)

Figure 6.1   Vaginal and cervical flora (all ×1000 magnified). (a) Normal: lactobacilli – seen as large Gram-positive rods – predominate. Squamous epithelial cells are Gram negative with a large amount of cytoplasm. (b) Candidiasis: there are speckled Gram-positive spores and long pseudohyphae visible. There are numerous polymorphs present and the bacterial flora is abnormal, resembling bacterial vaginosis. (c) Bacterial vaginosis: there is an overgrowth of anaerobic organisms, including *Gardnerella vaginalis* (small Gram-variable cocci), and a decrease in the numbers of lactobacilli. A 'clue cell' is seen. This is an epithelial cell covered with small bacteria so that the edge of the cell is obscured. (d) Trichomoniasis: an unstained 'wet mount' of vaginal fluid from a woman with *Trichomonas vaginalis* infection. There is a cone-shaped, flagellated organism in the centre, with a terminal spike and four flagella visible. In practice, the organism is identified under the microscope by movement, with amoeboid motion and its flagella waving.

Signs and symptoms 👁

- Vulval itching and soreness, thick curdy vaginal discharge, dyspareunia and dysuria.
- Vulval oedema, vulval excoriation, redness and erythema.
- Normal vaginal pH.

Diagnosis

It is important to confirm the diagnosis with a perineal and/or vaginal swab. Conditions such as contact dermatitis, allergic reactions and non-specific vaginal infections can present in a similar manner.

Testing can be done with a Gram stain or wet film examination and direct plating on to fungal media. Further testing to type the species may be required in recurrent or very severe cases as some species such as *C. krusei* can be resistant to some of the imidazoles, such as fluconazole (Figure 6.1b).

Predisposing factors

Pregnancy, high-dose combined oral contraceptive pill, immunosuppresion, broad spectrum antibiotics, diabetes mellitus, hormone replacement therapy and HIV-infected women have a higher predisposition to develop vulvovaginal candidiasis.

Treatment

Up to 30–40 per cent of asymptomatic women may have *C. albicans* grown on a vaginal swab. These women do not need treatment even if they are pregnant. There is no evidence of any adverse effects in pregnancy to either the mother or the baby if treated with topical imidazoles. However, the oral imidazoles are contraindicated in pregnancy.

General and supportive care

Women should be advised to avoid using any soaps, perfumes and synthetic underwear.

The high-dose oestrogen combined oral contraceptive pill should be changed to a lower-dose pill. If there are persistent or recurrent symptoms, consideration should be given to change to a progesterone-only contraception. Check blood sugars to rule out undiagnosed diabetes mellitus and if present good glycaemic control should be the aim. Avoid recurrent courses of broad spectrum antibiotics.

The treatment of vulvovaginal candidiasis can be based on whether the infection is uncomplicated, complicated or severe and recurrent.

Uncomplicated infection

Azoles/imidazoles are the mainstay of the treatment. They can either be used either as a local topical application (pessaries/creams) or oral preparations. There are several types of imidazoles with similar efficacy with a cure rate of over 80 per cent. The treatment is usually based on the preference of the physician, local availability and costs.

The common imidazoles are clotrimazole, econazole and miconazole. Other antifungals, such as nystatin cream or pessary, can also be used. The medication can be taken as a single pessary treatment or a course of pessaries for a few days at a lower dose. The commonly prescribed medication is clotrimazole, which can be taken as single 500 mg pessary or a course of a 100 mg pessary over 6 days.

Oral imidazoles, such as fluconazole, are given as a single dose at 150 mg or itraconazole 200 mg twice a day for 1 day. However, these are contraindicated in pregnancy.

There is no evidence to treat the asymptomatic male partner.

Complicated infection

Commonly seen in acute severe infection in pregnancy, women with diabetes mellitus or with immunosuppression conditions or therapy. The topical treatment in such cases can be extended to up to 2 weeks.

Recurrent infection

Recurrent infection is defined as at least four episodes of infection per year and/or a positive microscopy of moderate to heavy growth of *C. albicans*. In such cases, the principle of treatment would be an induction regimen to treat the acute episode followed by a maintenance regimen to treat further recurrences. Commonly fluconazole 150 mg is given in three doses orally every 72 hours followed by a maintenance dose of 150 mg weekly for six months. There is a 90 per cent cure rate at six months and 40 per cent at one year with this regimen. Oral imidazoles cannot be used in pregnancy but a topical imidazole can be used for 2 weeks for induction followed by a weekly dose of clotrimazole 500 mg for possibly 6–8 weeks. There are no trials to indicate the duration of therapy in such cases.

Other therapies

There is no evidence to support the use of oral/vaginal lactobacillus or the dietary intake of carbohydrates or yeasts to treat vulvovaginal candidiasis.

Trichomonas vaginalis

Trichomonas is a flagellate protozoan and can cause severe vulvovaginitis. It is usually sexually transmitted and commonly recurrences occur if the male partner is not simultaneously treated. It can also cause urinary tract infection.

Signs and symptoms
• Vulval soreness and itching
• Foul smelling vaginal discharge, sometimes frothy yellowish green in nature.
• Dysuria and abdominal discomfort
• Asymptomatic carriers
• Appearances of strawberry cervix due to the presence of punctate haemorrhages.

Diagnosis

Microscopy of vaginal discharge and culture in Finnberg–Whittington or Diamond's medium. Wet mount, where the discharge is mixed with saline and examined under the microscope, may show the motile protozoal organism with the typical flagellae. This is sensitive in diagnosing between 60 and 70 per cent of cases (Figure 6.1d).

Management

Both partners should be treated and both should be screened for other sexually transmitted infections.

Drug treatment

Metronidazole in a single oral dose of 2 g, or 400 mg twice daily, is a very effective with cure rates of up to 95 per cent. Single-dose regimens are more compliant and can be cheaper. Tinidazole in a single oral dose of 2 g is equally effective, but can cost more.

Treatment failures occur if the partner has not been treated, failure of compliance of the medication due to side effects, or resistance develops to the treatment. In such cases, the history should be reviewed, the route of administration changed (rectal rather than oral) or in some cases higher doses of metronidazole given. It is also thought that there may be some vaginal organisms which may reduce the potency of metronidazole, and treating the patient with some broad spectrum antibiotics may actually improve the response.

Bacterial vaginosis

Bacterial vaginosis is a common condition characterized by the presence of foul-smelling vaginal discharge with no obvious inflammation. It occurs due to the growth and increase in anaerobic species with simultaneous reduction in the lactobacilli in the vaginal flora causing an increase in the vaginal pH making it more alkaline (4.5 to 7.0). The common species involved are *Gardnerella vaginalis*, *Mycoplasma hominis*, *Bacteroides* spp. and *Mobilincus* spp. *Gardnerella* spp. are commonly isolated in women with no clinical signs of infection, so the diagnosis should be carefully considered.

Signs and symptoms

- Fishy malodorous vaginal discharge
- Asymptomatic carriers
- More prominent during and following menstruation
- Creamy or greyish-white vaginal discharge commonly adherent to the wall of the vagina.

Diagnostic features

Amsel criteria

1 Presence of clue cells on microscopic examination. Clue cells are epithelial cells which are covered with bacteria giving a characteristic stippled appearance on examination.
2 Creamy greyish white discharge which is seen on naked eye examination.
3 Vaginal pH of more than 4.5.
4 Release of a characteristic fishy odour on addition of alkali: 10 per cent potassium hydroxide.

There should be at least three criteria for diagnosing bacterial vaginosis using this Amsel criteria (Figure 6.1c).

Other criteria based on Gram staining of the vaginal discharge can also be used:

Hay/Ison criteria

Grade 1. Normal: Lactobacillus predominate.

Grade 2. Intermediate: Lactobacillus seen with the presence of *Gardnerella* and/or *Mobiluncus* spp.

Grade 3. Bacterial vaginosis: Lactobacilli absent or markedly reduced with predominance of *Gardnerella* and/or *Mobiluncus* spp.

Nugent criteria

Based on the proportion of anaerobic species giving a quantitative score between 0 and 10.

Less than 4: Normal

4 to 6: Intermediate

More than 6: Bacterial vaginosis

Management

Metronidazole either orally or as a gel is a simple and effective form of treatment. It is given in an oral dose of 400 mg twice a day for 5 days or a single dose of 2 g. Alternatively, it can be used as a local intravaginal gel (0.75 per cent) usually applied at night for between 5 and 7 days.

Clindamycin 300 mg twice daily or a topical vaginal cream (2 per cent) is also effective in treatment, however it is more expensive. There are also reports of damage to condoms and development of psuedomembranous colitis with clindamycin. However, the drug is more effective in treating the different anaerobic species when compared to metronidazole.

Pregnancy and bacterial vaginosis

Presence of bacterial vaginosis in the first trimester can lead to late second trimester miscarriages and preterm labour with its associated complications. Women with a previous history of second trimester loss or preterm delivery should have a vaginal swab performed in early pregnancy and if bacterial vaginosis is detected, it should be actively treated in the early second trimester of pregnancy. Metronidazole is safe to use in pregnancy, however, large or prolonged doses should be avoided.

Gonorrhoea

Gonorrhoea is a sexually transmitted disease caused by the Gram-negative diplococcus *Neisseria gonorrhoea*. It has affinity to infect the mucous membranes of the genital tract infecting cuboidal and columnar epithelium seen in the endocervical and urethral mucosa. It can also infect the rectal and oropharyngeal mucous membrane during anal and oral intercourse. There has been a gradual decline in the incidence of gonorrhoea and this could be the result of earlier detection and treatment. However, many women and their partners are asymptomatic carriers.

Sexually transmitted coinfection with *Chlamydia* and *Trichomonas* are common and can provoke more pronounced infection. These may lead to ascending infection causing endometritis, endosalpingitis and pelvic inflammatory disease.

Signs and symptoms

- Asymptomatic
- Increased vaginal discharge with lower abdominal/pelvic pain
- Dysuria with urethral discharge
- Proctitis with rectal bleeding, discharge and pain
- Endocervical mucopurulent discharge and contact bleeding
- Mucopurulent urethral discharge
- Pelvic tenderness with cervical excitation.

Diagnostic tests

- Gram staining: visualization of Gram-negative intracellular diplococci (Figure 6.2)

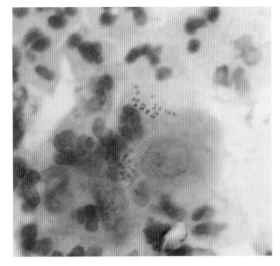

Figure 6.2 Vaginal and cervical flora (×1000 magnified). A Gram-stained smear of cervical secretions showing polymorphs and Gram-negative intracellular diplococci. This appearance is highly suggestive of gonorrhoea.

- Culture medium using an agar medium containing antimicrobials to reduce growth of other organisms
- Nucleic acid amplification tests (NAATs)
- Nucleic acid hybridization tests

Endocervical swabs should be taken and if symptomatic, swabs from the rectum and pharynx should also be included. The NAATs can test samples taken from the urine and low vagina.

Treatment

It is important to screen both partners and refer them to a genitourinary medicine (GUM) clinic. Contact tracing should be encouraged if there is exposure to multiple partners. They should be counselled regarding the long-term implications of the infections leading to chronic pelvic pain, tubal infection and subfertility.

Antibiotic treatment

Cephalosporins are the mainstay of treatment. There is emerging evidence of resistance of the organism to penicillin, ciprofloxacin and tetracycline, most likely due to mutations in the organisms. It is not necessary to repeat the swabs if there is certainty that the recommended medication has been taken. However, if there is any doubt of compliance, if the symptoms persist or there is a suspicion of resistance, then the swabs should be repeated within the week following treatment to check for complete cure.

The commonly prescribed antibiotics are:

- Single oral dose of cefixime 400 mg
- Single intramuscular dose of ceftriaxone 250 mg
- Single intramuscular dose of spectinomycin 2 g
- Single oral dose of ciprofloxacin 500 mg or ofloxacin 400 mg
- Ampicillin 2 g or amoxycillin 1 g with probenecid 2 gm as a single oral dose.

In pregnancy, it is safe to use the penicillins and cephalosporins, but tetracycline and ciprofloxacin/ofloxacin should be avoided.

Genitourinary chlamydia

Chlamydia is an obligate intracellular bacterium affecting the columnar epithelium of the genital tract. It causes one of the most common sexually transmitted infections. In the majority of cases, it is asymptomatic with slow and insidious infection leading to detrimental effects on the female genital tract. About 5–10 per cent of women below the age of 24 years are thought to carry the infection and there is ongoing reinfection and transmission due the asymptomatic nature of the disease. The UK Government has launched a national chlamydial screening programme as a result of the increasing incidence of the infection.

There are several serovars of chlamydia: A–C infect the conjunctiva causing trachoma and D–K infect the genitourinary system. Other chlamydia species, such as psittaci and pneumonia, infect the lungs causing pneumonia. There is a lymphogranuloma venereum strain (L1–L3) which can cause rectal infection and proctitis.

Pathophysiology

Infection occurs due to elementary bodies which enter the cells through specific receptors. Once inside, they form inclusion bodies which divide rapidly by binary fission. These then reform into elementary bodies and get released from the cell. This destroys the cell and the damage that occurs is due to the inflammatory response to the infection.

Signs and symptoms

- Asymptomatic
- Vaginal discharge and lower abdominal pain
- Postcoital bleeding
- Intermenstrual bleeding
- Mucopurulent cervical discharge with contact bleeding
- Dysuria with urethral discharge.

Complications

- Pelvic inflammatory disease
- Perihepatitis: Fitz–Hugh–Curtis syndrome
- Neonatal conjunctivitis and pneumonia
- Adult conjunctivitis
- Reiter's syndrome: reactive arthritis

Diagnostic tests

- Nucleic acid amplification technique: >90 per cent sensitive, should replace the old enzyme immunoassays (recommended by the Department of Health), should be used in all medicolegal cases and testing twice should improve the specificity of the test.
- Aptima Combo 2 and BD Probetec are the recommended tests for chlamydial infection.
- Real-time polymerase chain reaction
- Culture is expensive with limited availability. It has a 100 per cent specificity, however, is only around 60 per cent sensitive, hence not routinely recommended.

Screening and opportunistic testing

- Partners of patients diagnosed or suspected with infection
- History of chlamydia in the last year
- Patients attending GUM clinics
- Patients with two or more partners within 12 months
- Women undergoing termination of pregnancy
- History of other sexually transmitted infection and HIV.

Treatment

General advice

- Avoid intercourse, including oral and rectal, before treatment of both partners is complete.

- Use of condoms should be encouraged to prevent reinfection and other STIs.
- Retesting if any doubt about complete treatment. Test of cure should be performed a minimum of 5 weeks after initiation of treatment.
- Test of cure should be routine in pregnancy.
- Contact tracing of all partners when possible.
- A follow-up interview which could also include a telephonic consultation within 2–4 weeks.
- If change of partner, retesting between three to 12 months is recommended.

Antibiotic treatment

- Doxycycline 100 mg orally twice a day × 7days
- Azithromycin 1 g orally in a single dose, recommended treatment in pregnancy
- Erythromycin 500 mg orally four times a day × 7 days
- Amoxicillin 500 mg three times a day × 7 days
- Ofloxacin 200 mg orally twice a day or 400 mg once a day × 7 days.

Upper genital infection

Pelvic inflammatory disease

Pelvic inflammatory disease is characterized by inflammation and infection arising from the endocervix leading to endometritis, salpingitis, oophoritis, pelvic peritonitis and subsequently formation of tubo-ovarian and pelvic abscesses. Chlamydial and gonococcal infections are commonly implicated, however, other organisms, such as bacterial vaginosis, may be identified.

Pathophysiology

Once the infection has ascended to the upper genital tract, the Fallopian tubes are commonly damaged. There is inflammation of the mucosal lining which, if progressive, will destroy the cilia within the Fallopian tube followed by scarring in the tubal lumen. This can cause pocketing within the lumen with partial obstruction and thus predispose to ectopic pregnancy. In severe infection, mucopurulent discharge exudes through the fimbrial end of the Fallopian tube causing peritoneal inflammation. This can lead to scarring and

adhesion formation between the pelvic structures. It can affect the ovary and form a tubo-ovarian abscess with distortion of the anatomy. Infections are usually contained by the omentum and frequently omental adhesions are seen in the areas affected. Chlamydia and gonorrhoea can also cause perihepatitis leading to adhesions between the liver and the peritoneal surface. This gives a typical violin string appearance at laparoscopy and is known as the Fitz–Hugh–Curtis syndrome (Figure 6.3).

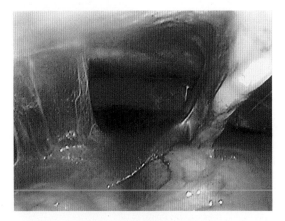

Figure 6.3 Fitz Hugh Curtis Syndrome showing perihepatic adhesions (typical violin string appeareance).

Signs and symptoms

- Abdominal, pelvic pain and dyspareunia
- Mucopurulent vaginal discharge
- Pyrexia (>38°C)
- Heavy/intermenstrual bleeding
- Pelvic tenderness and cervical excitation during examination
- Tender adnexal or palpable pelvic mass
- Generalized sepsis in severe and systemic infection
- Tubal damage leading to tubal occlusion, abscess and hydrosalpinx (Figures 6.4–6.7).

Diagnosis

Based on clinical findings:

- Raised white cell count (neutrophilia suggestive of acute inflammatory process)
- Reduced white cell count (neutropenia in severe infections)

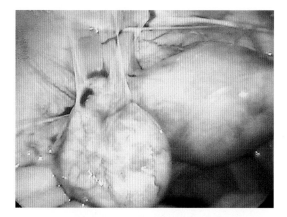

Figure 6.4   Peritubal adhesions of the left Fallopian tube.

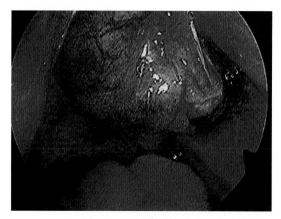

Figure 6.5   Left Fallopian tube with terminal hydrosalpinx.

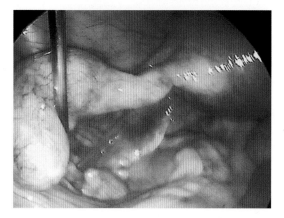

Figure 6.6   Left Fallopian tube hydrosalpinx.

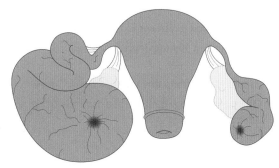

Figure 6.7   Large hydrosalpinx of the left Fallopian tube with a smaller hydrosalpinx on the right side.

- Raised C reactive protein and ESR (erythrocyte sedimentation rate)
- Adnexal masses on ultrasound
- Laparoscopy is the gold standard to give a definitive diagnosis, however, in mild cases it may not be very obvious.

Treatment

Depending on the severity of the infection, patients with mild/moderate disease can be managed on an outpatient basis with easy access to hospital admission if the infection becomes more severe. An intrauterine contraceptive device, if present, should be removed and alternative emergency contraception or other modes of contraception (combined pill, oral/parenteral progesterone) should be offered. A

pregnancy test should be done in all cases to rule out ectopic pregnancy.

There are several differing antibiotic regimes that are used; however, the following is recommended by the RCOG Green Top Guideline (2008) which is evidence based.

- Mild/moderate infection (outpatient treatment)
  - Oral ofloxacin 400 mg twice a day + oral metronidazole 400 mg twice a day × 14 days
  - Ceftriaxone 250 mg single intramuscular injection + oral doxycycline 100 mg twice a day + oral metronidazole 400 mg twice a day × 14 days
  - Single intramuscular dose of ceftriaxone 250 mg + azithromycin 1 g/week × 2 weeks. The data supporting the use of azithromycin are limited and should not be used in isolation.

This type of triple antibiotic therapy is important to provide a broad spectrum of cover as PID is caused by multiple organisms, in addition to chlamydia and gonococcus.

- Hospitalization and parenteral therapy: patients should be admitted to the hospital when there is evidence of:
  - Severe infection
  - Adnexal masses suspicious of abscess
  - Generalized sepsis
  - Poor/inadequate response to oral treatment
  - Severe pelvic/abdominal pain requiring strong analgesics.

Principles of treatment

- Adequate supportive care
- Strict watch on fluid balance
- Parenteral antibiotics
  - Ceftriaxone 2 g i.v. + i.v./oral doxycycline 100 mg twice daily + i.v. metronidazole 500 mg twice daily. This should be continued until the patient gets clinically better which is usually within 24 hours, following which the antibiotics should be changed to oral therapy for 14 days.
  - Clindamycin 900 mg i.v. three times daily + gentamycin i.v. (loading dose 2 mg/kg followed by 1.5 mg/kg three times a day) followed by either clindamycin 450 mg four times daily or oral doxycycline twice daily + oral metronidazole 400 mg daily for 14 days.
  - Ofloxacin i.v. 400 mg twice daily + metronidazole i.v. three times a day × 14 days.

- In pregnancy, a combination of cefotaxime + azithromycin + metronidazole should be used. Doxycycline, gentamycin and ofloxacin should be avoided.

Surgical treatment

In patients with a pelvic abscess or patients not responding to therapy, a laparoscopy is warranted. This may also exclude other causes of pain, such as appendicitis, endometriosis or ovarian pathology. The usual treatment would involve drainage of the abscess and sometimes the affected tube/ovary may have to be removed.

Patient counselling

- Partner and other sexual contacts should be screened.
- There is a risk of reinfection if the partner is not treated.
- Use of barrier contraception will reduce the risk of further recurrences.
- Risks of tubal damage leading to subfertility, ectopic pregnancy and chronic pelvic pain which increases with further episodes of infection.
- Prompt and early treatment will reduce the risk of subfertility.
- Seek early medical advice if pregnant, due to the risk of an ectopic pregnancy.

Other infections

Other infections are described in Table 6.1.

Table 6.1   Other genital infections

Infection	Causative organism	Clinical features	Diagnosis	Treatment
Primary herpes	Herpes simplex virus type I (usually oral) or type II (usually genital)	Painful vesicles and multiple ulcerations on vulva Retention of urine	Swab from ulcer Serum from vesicle Virus seen on electron microscopy Culture	Acyclovir 200 mg five times/day Famciclovir Valaciclovir Analgesics and local anaesthetic gels
Genital warts	Human papillomavirus HPV 6 and 11 HPV 16 and 18 linked to cervical cancer	Warty lesions on the vulva, vagina, cervix and perianal area Also seen around mouth, lips and larynx if orogenital contact	Clinical examination Histology of removed wart Seen on cervical smear and colposcopy	Podophyllin local application twice a week Surgical excision Laser Cryotherapy
Syphilis	*Treponema pallidum*	Primary syphilis: Painless ulcer/ulcers on vulva, vagina or cervix Enlarged groin/inguinal lymph nodes Secondary syphilis: maculopapular rash on palms and soles	TPPA: *Treponema pallidum* particle agglutination TPHA: *Treponema pallidum* haemagglutination assay FTA: Fluorescent treponemal antibody	Penicillin mainstay of treatment Procaine penicillin 1.2 MU daily i.m. × 12 days Benzathine penicillin 2.4 MU i.m. repeated after 7 days

Infection	Causative organism	Clinical features	Diagnosis	Treatment
		Mucous membrane ulcers	Dark field illumination: serum from base of ulcer + saline taken and seen under the microscope. Spiral organisms with characteristic movements are diagnostic	Doxycycline 100 mg bd × 14 days
		Generalized lymphadenopathy, arthritis		Erythromycin 500 mg qds × 14 days
		Neurosyphilis: meningitis, stroke, tabes dorsalis		
		Cardiovascular: aortic aneurysm		
		Congenital syphilis: intrauterine death, interstitial keratitis, VIII nerve deafness, abnormal teeth		
Genital tuberculosis	*Mycobacterium tuberculosis*	Usually following pulmonary tuberculosis through blood and lymphatics	Histological confirmation from endometrium and Fallopian tube	Rifampicin
		Amenorrhoea (affects endometrium)	Mantoux test	Isoniazid
		Infertility (affects tube)	Heaf test	Pyrazinamide
		Acute/chronic pelvic pain	Chest x-ray	Treatments can last from six to 12 months
		Frozen pelvis due to severe multiple adhesions		
Chancroid	*Haemophilus ducreyi*	Painful shallow multiple ulcers	Specialized culture	Single oral dose of azithromycin 2 g

Infection	Causative organism	Clinical features	Diagnosis	Treatment
		Regional lymphadenopathy with suppuration	Isolation of Ducrey's bacillus on biopsy	Ceftriaxone Erythromycin
Granuloma inguinale	*Klebsiella granulomatosis*	Painless nodule	Donovan bodies: intracellular inclusions seen in phagocytes or histiocytes	Erythromycin
Donovanosis		Painful ulcers Local tissue destruction		Tetracycline Streptomycin

CASE HISTORY

A 29-year-old woman presents to the emergency gynaecology unit with a 5-day history of lower abdominal and pelvic pain which has got progressively worse over the last 24 hours. She also feels generally unwell with chills and rigors. She has had several partners and was found to have *Chlamydia* a few years ago. She is not sure whether she completed the whole course of treatment and did not go back to get tested. She does not use any form of contraception and has had unprotected intercourse recently.

On examination, she looks very unwell. She has a raised temperature at 38°C and is tachycardic. She is very tender on abdominal examination with guarding. On speculum examination, the cervix appears inflamed with profuse mucopurulent discharge. A high vaginal swab, endocervical swab and a urethral swab are taken. On pelvic examination, there is marked cervical tenderness. She is also generally tender to palpate throughout the pelvis and is unable to tolerate the examination. A pregnancy test is negative.

The clinical diagnosis is suggestive of acute pelvic inflammatory disease with pelvic peritonitis. She is admitted and started with intravenous antibiotics (ceftriaxone + metronidazole) and oral doxycycline. She is also supported with intravenous fluids, analgesics and regular paracetamol. A pelvic ultrasound shows the possibility of an adnexal mass with some free fluid in the pelvis. She continues to be unwell with a raised temperature even after 24 hours of antibiotics. Thus, a decision is taken to perform a laparoscopy. At the operation, she is found to have a 7-cm enlarged tubo-ovarian abscess and marked inflammation of the uterus and other tube. The abscess is drained and the patient markedly improves after the surgery. She is found to have chlamydia on the endocervical swab with anaerobes on the high vaginal swab. She improves over the course of a few days and is treated with oral antibiotics for 2 weeks. She is counselled regarding the implications of the infection and is encouraged to contact her present and previous partners for testing, of whom one tested positive for *Chlamydia* and was subsequently treated.

Key Points

- Acute PID can be life threatening.

- Other differential diagnosis should be kept in mind (ectopic pregnancy, appendicitis).

- Detailed sexual history should be taken.

- Incomplete treatment of sexually transmitted infections should be avoided as there is a high chance of recurrence.

- Surgical treatment should not be delayed if patient's general condition is not improving with conservative treatment.

- Thorough counselling regarding the implications of infection with regards to subfertility and risk of ectopic pregnancy should be offered.

- All attempts to contact present and previous partners should be encouraged and made.

- Patients should be advised to use barrier contraception until the infection is completely cured. Test of cure should be done.

Additional reading and websites

Bignell C. *National guideline on the diagnosis and treatment of gonorrhoea in adults.* London: BASHH, 2005.

British Association for Sexual Health and HIV. BASHH guidelines. Available from www.bashh.org.

Hay P. *National guideline for the management of bacterial vaginosis.* London: BASHH, 2006.

Horner P. *UK national guideline for the management of genital tract infection with Chlamydia trachomatis.* London: BASHH, 2006.

Royal College of Obstetricians and Gynaecologists. Green Top Guideline No. 32. *Management of acute pelvic inflammatory disease.* London: RCOG, 2008.

Royal College of Obstetricians and Gynaecologists. RCOG Green Top guidelines. Available from www.rcog.org.uk.

Scottish Intercollegiate Guidelines Network. *Management of genital Chlamydia trachomatis infection*, SIGN 109. Edinburgh: SIGN, 2009.

Scottish Intercollegiate Guidelines Network. SIGN guidelines. Available from www.sign.ac.uk.

White D, Robertson C. *United Kingdom national guideline on the management of vulvovaginal candidiasis.* London: BASHH, 2007.

OVERVIEW

Contraception is provided entirely free of charge in the UK. A wide range of methods exists and people will use different methods at different stages of their lives. When women no longer wish to conceive, they may consider a sterilization method, although long-acting reversible contraception is increasingly encouraged as an alternative to sterilization. Despite the widespread availability of contraception, unintended pregnancy is still common in the UK and some women will choose to have an abortion, by either a medical or surgical technique.

Contraception

Around the world, contraception has been used, in one form or another, for thousands of years. Many women will use it for extremely long periods of time in their reproductive lifespan; the average age of first intercourse in the UK is 16 years and the mean age of menopause is 51 years. People will use different types of contraception at different stages in their lives and there is no one method that will suit everyone. Women tend to take most of the responsibility for contraception, but the needs and wishes of the male partners should also be considered if a method is to be used effectively.

There is no perfect method of contraception and each method will have a balance of advantages and disadvantages. The characteristics of the ideal contraceptive method would be:

- highly effective;
- no side effects or risks;
- cheap;
- independent of intercourse and requires no regular action on the part of the user;
- non-contraceptive benefits;
- acceptable to all cultures and religions;
- easily distributed and administrated by non-healthcare personnel.

Classification of contraception

- Combined hormonal contraception
  - The pill
  - Patches
  - The vaginal ring
- Progestogen-only preparations
  - Progestogen-only pills
  - Injectables
  - Subdermal implants
- Hormonal emergency contraception
- Intrauterine contraception
  - Copper intrauterine device (IUD)
  - Hormone-releasing intrauterine system (IUS)
- Barrier methods
  - Condoms
  - Female barriers
  - Coitus interruptus
  - Natural family planning
- Sterilization
  - Female sterilization
  - Vasectomy

Use of contraception in the UK

Contraceptive usage is very high in the UK and more than 95 per cent of women in the UK who do not want to become pregnant will use contraception. In contrast to most other countries, contraception is provided entirely free of charge for the user in the UK. The user also has a choice of where to obtain contraception; it is available from both general practitioners and from community contraceptive clinics.

Patterns of use of methods of contraception in the UK are listed in Table 7.1. Some couples may use more than one method at the same time, for example taking the oral contraceptive pill in conjunction with using condoms.

Table 7.1   Patterns of contraceptive use in the UK 2008

Method of contraception	Use (%)
Combined oral contraceptive pill	36
Condoms	28
Intrauterine contraception (copper devices and Mirena®)	7
Injectable medroxyprogesterone acetate (DMPA or Depo-Provera®)	4
Withdrawal (coitus interruptus)	4
Natural family planning	3
Implanon®	2
Diaphragms	<1
Sterilization	11
Vasectomy	13

Failure rates

All methods of contraception can occasionally fail and some are much more effective than others. Failure rates are traditionally expressed as the number of failures per 100 woman-years (HWY), i.e. the number of pregnancies if 100 women were to use the method for one year. The efficacy rates of the various contraceptive methods are listed in Table 7.2.

The effectiveness of a method depends on two factors:

1 how it works;

2 how easy it is to use.

Failure rates for some methods vary considerably, largely because of the potential for failure caused

Table 7.2   Effectiveness of contraceptive methods

Method of contraception	Failure rate per 100 woman years
Combined oral contraceptive pill	0.1–1
Progestogen-only pill	1–3
Depo-Provera®	0.1–2
Implanon®	0.1
Copper IUD	1–2
Mirena®	0.5
Male condom	2–5
Diaphragm	1–15
Natural family planning	2–3
Vasectomy	0.02
Female sterilization	0.13

by poor use (user failure) rather than an intrinsic failure of the method itself. Methods which prevent ovulation are usually highly effective because if there is no egg then fertilization simply cannot occur. However, if, for example, pills are forgotten, then breakthrough ovulation can occur and failure rates are higher. Methods which require no regular need for the user to remember to do anything, for example an intrauterine device or Implanon®, are generally much more effective than methods which rely on the user to do something regularly.

Compliance and continuation

Many people use contraception incorrectly and inconsistently. Studies looking at pill use report nearly half of all women missing at least one pill per packet and a quarter missing two pills. The contraceptive injection is highly effective, but women can forget to attend for their repeat injection. Methods which require correct use with every act of intercourse have the highest failure rates, for example condoms, natural family planning.

Women are often quick to stop contraception because of perceived side effects, such as weight gain or mood change. Methods which need to be inserted or removed by health professionals tend to have better continuation rates as they cannot be easily abandoned in the heat of the moment.

Increasing the uptake of implants, injectables and intrauterine contraception (long-acting reversible contraception or LARC) is a key strategy in the UK to reduce unplanned pregnancy.

Contraindications

Although contraception is generally extremely safe, some methods do have very rare but serious risks. It is important to establish any factors in the medical history that could contraindicate a particular method. No method is contraindicated by age alone. The World Health Organization (WHO) has published clear guidelines on assessing the criteria for contraceptive use which have been adapted for UK practice (Table 7.3). This document is widely used in clinical practice (see Additional reading section).

Table 7.3   UK Medical Eligibility Criteria for contraceptive use

Category	Classification of condition	Use of the method in practice
1	No restriction for the use of the method	Use in any circumstance
2	The advantages of using the method generally outweigh the theoretical or proven risks	Generally use
3	The theoretical or proven risks usually outweigh the advantages of using the method; requires careful clinical judgement and access to clinical services	Not usually recommended unless other, more appropriate, methods are not available or not acceptable
4	Represents an unacceptable health risk if the contraceptive method is used	Do not use

Non-contraceptive health benefits

Some methods of contraception offer significant benefits over and above their contraceptive effect which can be important factors in contraceptive choice. Condoms prevent sexually transmitted infections. Many methods containing hormones, particularly the Mirena®, help heavy or painful periods. Some women who do not need contraception choose to use hormonal preparations for these benefits alone.

The combined pill protects against both ovarian and endometrial cancer. Condoms and diaphragms both protect against cervical cancer.

The contraceptive consultation

During the contraceptive consultation, there is often a great deal of information to discuss and not much time. The user needs to make an informed choice about which method to use. The discussion about a method needs to cover:

- mode of action;
- effectiveness;
- side effects or risks;
- benefits;
- how to use the method.

It is often helpful to give back-up written information. Contraceptive counselling is multidisciplinary and specialist nurses play an important role. Some methods of contraception are only available on prescription, whereas others can be used without ever having to seek medical advice.

Counselling about sexually transmitted infections (STI) and HIV risk reduction and prevention is an integral part of a comprehensive contraceptive consultation.

Combined hormonal contraception

Combined oral contraceptive pills

Combined oral contraception (COC) – 'the pill' – was first licensed in the UK in 1961 and its development marked a very significant milestone in contraception. It contains a combination of two hormones: a synthetic oestrogen and a progestogen (a synthetic derivative of progesterone).

Since COC was first introduced, the doses of both oestrogen and progestogen have been reduced dramatically, which has considerably improved its safety profile.

It is estimated that at least 200 million women worldwide have taken COC since it was first marketed, and there are currently around three million users in the UK alone.

A combined hormonal patch and a combined contraceptive vaginal ring (CCVR) are also available. They are discussed specifically below, but share most of the benefits and risks of combined oral contraception. A combined contraceptive injection which is given monthly is also licensed in some countries, but not the UK.

Combined oral contraception is easy to use and offers a very high degree of protection against pregnancy, with many other beneficial effects. It is mainly used by young, healthy women who wish a method of contraception that is independent of intercourse. For maximum effectiveness, COC should always be taken regularly at roughly the same time each day.

Mode of action

Combined oral contraception acts both centrally and peripherally.

- Inhibition of ovulation is by far the most important effect. Both oestrogen and progestogen suppress the release of pituitary follicle-stimulating hormone (FSH) and luteinizing hormone (LH), which prevents follicular development within the ovary and therefore ovulation.
- Peripheral effects include making the endometrium atrophic and hostile to implantation and altering cervical mucus to prevent sperm ascending into the uterine cavity.

Formulations

There are many different formulations and brands of COC (Figure 7.1) which increasingly offer different hormones, dosages and pill taking schedules. In practice, in the UK, many women will take the same basic formulation, although women from abroad may present requesting a much wider range of pills.

Oestrogens

Most modern preparations contain the oestrogen ethinyl estradiol (EE) in a daily dose of between 15 and 35 μg. Those containing lower dosages are associated with slightly poorer cycle control. Those containing higher daily dosages, for example 50 μg EE, are generally now only prescribed in special situations,

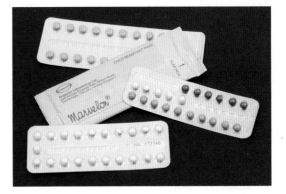

Figure 7.1 Combined oral contraceptive pill preparations.

discussed below. Higher dosages of oestrogen (above 50 μg EE) are strongly linked to increased risks of both arterial and venous thrombosis (see below). A new combined preparation contains the natural oestrogen, estradiol valerate, in place of synthetic EE, although it is not known if this confers any significant advantages.

Progestogens

Most COC contains progestogens that are classed as second or third generation. Second generation pills contain derivatives of norethindrone and levonorgestrel. The third generation pills include desogestrel, gestodene and norgestimate. Pills containing the newer progestogens, drospirenone and dienogest, are also available in the UK. A combined preparation licensed for the treatment of acne and hirsutism (but not contraception) contains the potent anti-androgen cyproterone acetate (Dianette®)

Regimens

Monophasic pills are almost always used and contain standard daily dosages of oestrogen and progestogen. Biphasic, triphasic or quadriphasic preparations have two, three or four incremental variations in hormone dose but are more complicated for women to use and have few real advantages.

Most brands contain 21 pills; one pill to be taken daily, followed by a 7-day pill-free interval (the traditional 21/7 model). There are also some every-day (ED) preparations that include seven placebo pills that are taken instead of having a pill-free interval. Newer brands, particularly from abroad, offer a wider combination of active pills and pill-free days with combinations such as 24/4, 84/7 and 365 (where a pill is taken daily without any breaks).

Contraindications

The UK Medical Eligibility criteria have helpful tables on the category 3 and 4 contraindications to COC (see Tables 7.4 and 7.5). Most of these relate to the side effects of sex steroid hormones on the cardiovascular and hepatic systems.

Women should ideally discontinue COC at least two months before any elective pelvic or leg surgery because of the risk of venous thromboembolism.

Side effects and risks

The vast majority of women tolerate COC well, with few problems. However, COC has effects throughout the entire body and a large number of potential side effects/risks exist. Common side effects are listed in Table 7.6 and, although often minor, frequently lead to early discontinuation. Many minor side effects will settle within a few months of starting COC.

The most important risks relate to cardiovascular disease, as detailed below.

Venous thromboembolism

COC increases risk of venous thromboembolism (VTE) three- to five-fold. Oestrogens (in COC, pregnancy and with hormone replacement therapy) alter blood clotting and coagulation in a way that induces a pro-thrombotic tendency, although the exact mechanism of this is poorly understood. The effect appears independent of dose of EE dose below 50 µg (but is significantly increased with higher dosages above this).

Table 7.4 UK Medical Eligibility Criteria 2006 category 4 conditions (absolute contraindications) for use of the combined oral contraceptive pill

Breastfeeding <6 weeks postpartum
Smoking ≥15 cigarettes/day and age ≥35
Multiple risk factors for cardiovascular disease
Hypertension: systolic pressure ≥160 or diastolic ≥100 mmHg
Hypertension with vascular disease
Current or history of deep-vein thrombosis/ pulmonary embolism
Major surgery with prolonged immobilization
Known thrombogenic mutations
Current or history of ischaemic heart disease
Current or history of stroke
Complicated valvular heart disease
Migraine with aura
Migraine without aura and age ≥35 (continuation)
Current breast cancer
Diabetes for ≥20 years or with severe vascular disease or with severe nephropathy, retinopathy or neuropathy
Active viral hepatitis
Severe cirrhosis
Benign or malignant liver tumours
Reproduced with permission from the Faculty of Sexual and Reproductive Healthcare, UK.

Table 7.5 UK Medical Eligibility Criteria 2006 category 3 conditions (relative contraindications) for use of the combined oral contraceptive pill

Multiple risk factors for arterial disease
Hypertension: systolic blood pressure 140–159 or diastolic pressure 90–99 mmHg, or adequately treated to below 140/90 mmHg
Some known hyperlipidaemias
Diabetes mellitus with vascular disease
Smoking (<15 cigarettes/day) and age ≥35 years
Obesity
Migraine, even without aura, and age ≥35 years
Breast cancer with >5 years without recurrence
Breastfeeding until six months postpartum
Postpartum and not breastfeeding until 21 days after childbirth
Current or medically treated gallbladder disease
History of cholestasis related to combined oral contraceptives
Mild cirrhosis
Taking rifampicin (rifampin) or certain anticonvulsants
Reproduced with permission from the Faculty of Sexual and Reproductive Healthcare, UK.

Table 7.6   Commonly reported side effects of COC

Common side effects of COC	
Central nervous system	Depressed mood
	Mood swings
	Headaches
	Loss of libido
Gastrointestinal	Nausea
	Perceived weight gain
	Bloatedness
Reproductive system	Breakthrough bleeding
	Increased vaginal discharge
Breasts	Breast pain
	Enlarged breasts
Miscellaneous	Chloasma (facial pigmentation which worsens with time on COC)
	Fluid retention
	Change in contact lens

The type of progestogen also affects the risk of VTE, with users of COC containing third-generation progestogens being twice as likely to sustain a VTE than those using older second-generation preparations. The absolute risk of an event with COC is very small but increased in the presence of an inherited thrombophilia. Women with a significant family history of VTE should be carefully assessed and tested for inherited thrombophilias prior to being prescribed COC.

The risks of VTE are:

- 5 per 100 000 for normal population;
- 15 per 100 000 for users of second-generation COC;
- 30 per 100 000 for users of third-generation COC;
- 60 per 100 000 for pregnant women.

Arterial disease

Arterial disease with COC is much less common than VTE but more serious. The risk of myocardial infarction and thrombotic stroke in young, healthy women using low-dose COC is extremely small.

However, cigarette smoking and high blood pressure will both increase the risk, and any woman who smokes must be advised to stop COC at the age of 35 years. Around 1 per cent of women taking COC will become significantly hypertensive and they should be advised to stop taking it.

Breast cancer

Advising women about the association between breast cancer and COC is very difficult. Most data do show a slight increase in the risk of developing breast cancer among current COC users (relative risk around 1.24). This is not of great significance to young women, as the background rate of breast cancer is very low at their age. However, for a woman in her forties or one with a strong family history, these are more relevant data, as their background rate of breast cancer is higher. Most data also show that any effect of COC on breast cancer risk has disappeared ten years after stopping COC.

Drug interactions

This can occur with enzyme-inducing agents, such as some anti-epileptic drugs. Higher dose estrogen pill combinations of 50 µg EE may need to be prescribed. Some broad-spectrum antibiotics can alter intestinal absorption of COC and reduce its efficacy. Additional contraceptive measures should therefore be recommended during antibiotic therapy and for 1 week thereafter.

Positive health benefits

Not all side effects of COC are unwanted! COC users generally have light, pain-free, regular bleeds and therefore COC can be used to treat heavy or painful periods. It can also improve premenstrual syndrome (PMS) and reduce the risk of pelvic inflammatory disease (PID). COC offers long-term protection against both ovarian and endometrial cancers. It can also be used as a treatment for acne.

Patient management

For a woman to take COC successfully there must be careful teaching and explanation of the method. Before COC is prescribed, a detailed past medical and family history should be taken and blood pressure checked (Figure 7.2). Routine weighing, breast and pelvic examinations are not required. Most women are given a three-month supply of COC in the first instance, and have 6–12-monthly reviews thereafter.

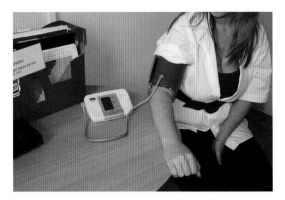

Figure 7.2 Monitoring blood pressure in a woman taking the combined oral contraceptive pill.

Woman need clear advice about what to do if they miss any pills (Figure 7.3).

Combined hormonal patches

A contraceptive transdermal patch containing oestrogen and progestogen is licensed in the UK and releases norelgestromin 150 mg and ethinylestradiol 20 mg per 24 hours (Figure 7.4). Patches are applied weekly for 3 weeks, after which there is a patch-free week. Contraceptive patches have the same risks and benefits as COC and, although they are relatively more expensive, may have better compliance.

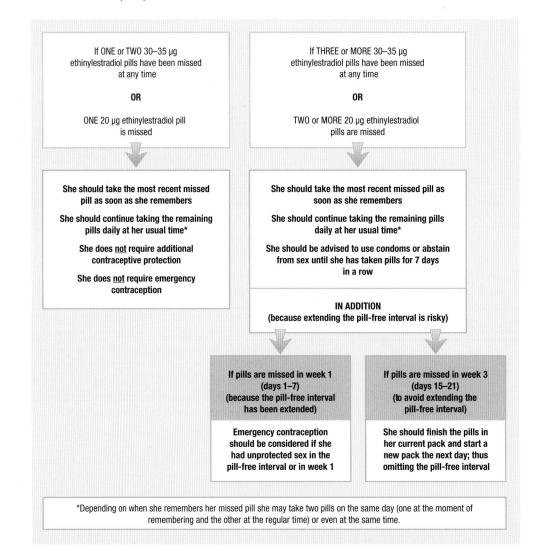

If ONE or TWO 30–35 µg ethinylestradiol pills have been missed at any time **OR** ONE 20 µg ethinylestradiol pill is missed	If THREE or MORE 30–35 µg ethinylestradiol pills have been missed at any time **OR** TWO or MORE 20 µg ethinylestradiol pills are missed
She should take the most recent missed pill as soon as she remembers. She should continue taking the remaining pills daily at her usual time*. She does **not** require additional contraceptive protection. She does **not** require emergency contraception	She should take the most recent missed pill as soon as she remembers. She should continue taking the remaining pills daily at her usual time*. She should be advised to use condoms or abstain from sex until she has taken pills for 7 days in a row

IN ADDITION
(because extending the pill-free interval is risky)

If pills are missed in week 1 (days 1–7) (because the pill-free interval has been extended)	If pills are missed in week 3 (days 15–21) (to avoid extending the pill-free interval)
Emergency contraception should be considered if she had unprotected sex in the pill-free interval or in week 1	She should finish the pills in her current pack and start a new pack the next day; thus omitting the pill-free interval

*Depending on when she remembers her missed pill she may take two pills on the same day (one at the moment of remembering and the other at the regular time) or even at the same time.

Figure 7.3 Algorithm for management of missed pills. Reproduced with permission from Faculty of Sexual and Reproductive Healthcare, Missed Pills Faculty Statement from the CEU. www.fsrh.org/admin/uploads/MissedPillRules%20.pdf.

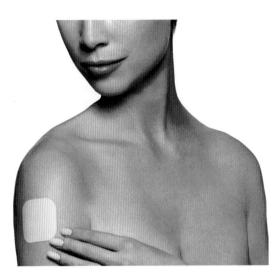

Figure 7.4 Combined contraceptive patch. Photograph courtesy of Janssen Cilag UK Ltd.

Combined hormonal vaginal rings

A combined contraceptive vaginal ring is licensed in the UK (Figure 7.5). It is made of latex-free plastic and has a diameter of 54 mm. It releases a daily dose of ethinyl estradiol 15 µg and etonorgestrel 120 µg. The ring is worn for 21 days and removed for 7 days, during which time a withdrawal bleed occurs. Insertion and removal of the ring is easy and it does not need to fit in any special place in the vagina. The cycle control is excellent and probably better than with COC. As with combined patches, the vaginal ring has the same risks and benefits as COC but is more expensive.

Progestogen-only contraception

Progestogen-only contraception avoids the risks and side effects of oestrogen.

The current methods of progestogen-only contraception are:

- progestogen-only pill, or 'mini-pill'
- subdermal implant (Implanon)
- injectables (Depo-Provera®, Noristerat®)
- hormone-releasing intrauterine system (Mirena) (see 'Intrauterine contraception' below).

All progestogen-only methods work by a local effect on cervical mucus (making it hostile to ascending sperm) and on the endometrium (making it thin and atrophic), thereby preventing implantation and sperm transport. The higher dose progestogen-only methods will also act centrally and inhibit ovulation, making them highly effective.

As they do not contain oestrogen, progestogen-only methods are extremely safe and can be used if a woman has cardiovascular risk factors, for example older women who smoke.

The common side effects of progestogen-only methods include:

- erratic or absent menstrual bleeding;
- simple, functional ovarian cysts;
- breast tenderness;
- acne.

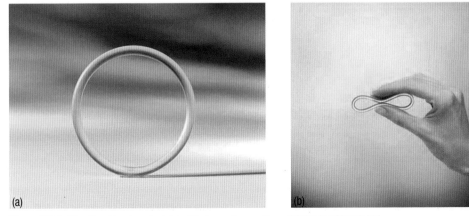

(a) (b)

Figure 7.5 (a,b) Combined vaginal ring. Photographs courtesy of Schering Plough Ltd.

Progestogen-only pills

The progestogen-only pill (POP) is ideal for women who like the convenience of pill taking but wish to avoid COC. It is taken every day without a break. Although the failure rate of the POP is greater than that of COC (see Table 7.2), it is ideal for women at times of lower fertility as detailed below. If the POP fails, there is a slightly higher risk of ectopic pregnancy.

There is only a small selection of brands in the UK (Figure 7.6) and they contain the second-generation progestogen norethisterone or norgestrel (or their derivatives) and the third-generation progestogen desogestrel. The dose of desogestrel in the POP Cerazette® inhibits ovulation in almost every cycle of use making it highly effective and the pill of choice for young women who cannot take the combined pill.

Particular indications for the POP include:

- breastfeeding;
- older age;
- cardiovascular risk factors, for example high blood pressure, smoking or diabetes.

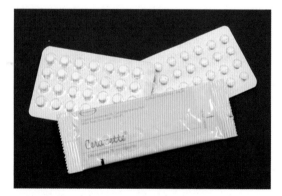

Figure 7.6   Progestogen-only pill preparations.

Injectable progestogens

Two injectable progestogens are marketed in the UK:

1 depot medroxyprogesterone acetate 150 mg (Depo-Provera/DMPA);

2 norethisterone enanthate 200 mg (Noristerat).

Most women choose Depo-Provera and each injection lasts for 12 weeks with a 2-week grace period

thereafter. Norethisterone enanthate only lasts for 8 weeks and is not nearly so widely used.

Depo-Provera is highly effective and it is given by deep intramuscular injection (Figure 7.7). Most women who use it develop very light or absent menstruation. Depo-Provera will improve PMS and can be used to treat menstrual problems such as painful or heavy periods. It is very useful for women who have difficulty remembering to take a pill regularly.

Depo-Provera causes low oestrogen levels and this is associated with loss of bone mineral density. It is not known if this translates into a higher risk of osteoporosis in later life. Bone density seems to recover when Depo-Provera is stopped. Women with pre-existing risk factors for osteoporosis should probably be advised not to use Depo-Provera in the long term.

Particular side effects of Depo-Provera include:

- weight gain of around 2–3 kg in the first year of use;
- delay in return of fertility – it may take around six months longer to conceive compared to a woman who stops COC;
- persistently irregular periods; most women become amenorrhoeic.

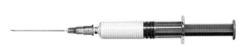

Figure 7.7   Depo-Provera.

Subdermal implants

Implanon consists of a single silastic rod (Figure 7.8) that is inserted subdermally under local anaesthetic into the upper arm (Figure 7.9). It releases the progestogen etonogestrel 25–70 mg daily (the dose released decreases with time), which is metabolized to the third-generation progestogen desogestrel. It lasts for three years and thereafter can be easily removed and a further implant inserted if requested.

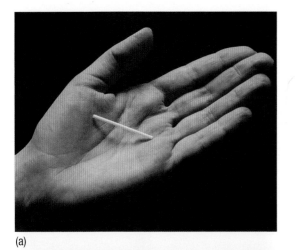

(a)

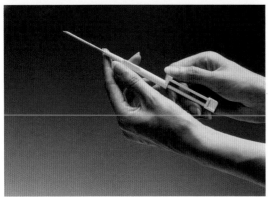

(b)

Figure 7.8 (a,b)   Implanon.

Implanon is particularly useful for women who have difficulty remembering to take a pill and who want highly effective long-term contraception. There is a rapid return of fertility when it is removed.

Women should be carefully counselled about the change in bleeding patterns with Implanon. Irregular bleeding is very common and is the major reason for early discontinuation.

Healthcare professionals need special training for Implanon insertion and removal. Removal can be difficult if the implant is inserted too deeply. If the implant cannot be palpated then it can be localized with high frequency ultrasound.

Intrauterine contraception

Modern intrauterine contraception is highly effective and is becoming increasingly popular in the UK. It is ideal for women who want a medium- to long-term method of contraception independent of intercourse and where regular compliance is not required. Intrauterine contraception protects against both intrauterine and ectopic pregnancy but, if pregnancy occurs, there is a higher chance than normal that it will be ectopic.

Fitting of an intrauterine contraception is performed by trained healthcare personnel and is a brief procedure associated with mild to moderate discomfort. A fine thread is left protruding from the cervix into the vagina and the IUD can be removed in due course by traction on this thread (Figure 7.10).

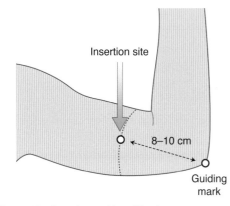

Figure 7.9   Insertion position of Implanon.

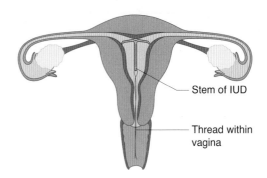

Figure 7.10   Intrauterine device (IUD) in the uterine cavity.

Types

Copper intrauterine device

Copper-bearing devices are available in various shapes and sizes. They cause much less menstrual disruption than the older plastic devices which are now no longer available. Most copper IUDs are licensed for ten years of use, although the small devices may only be for five years. The more copper a device has, the more effective it is. The modern 'banded' device has copper on the stem and copper sleeves on the arms (Figure 7.11).

An IUD without a frame, which consists of six copper beads on a prolene thread, has been developed and is anchored into the uterine fundus with a knot (GyneFix®).

Hormone releasing intrauterine system (Mirena)

Hormone-releasing devices have also been developed (Figure 7.12). The Mirena has a capsule containing levonorgestrel around its stem which releases a daily dose of 20 µg of hormone. It is associated with a dramatic reduction in menstrual blood loss and is licensed for contraception, the treatment of heavy menstrual bleeding and as part of a hormone replacement therapy (HRT) regimen.

The characteristics of the IUD and Mirena are compared in Table 7.7.

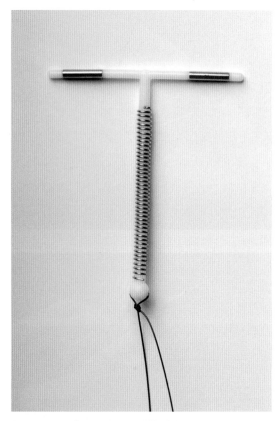

Figure 7.11   Copper bearing IUD with copper on stem and arms. Photograph courtesy of Durbin Ltd.

Table 7.7   Copper IUD and Mirena

	Copper IUD	Mirena
Failure rate in first year of use	0.8%	0.1%
Mode of action	Toxic effect on both sperm and egg, i.e. acting prior to fertilization	Local hormonal effect on the cervical mucus and endometrium
Duration of use	10 years	5 years
Effect on menstrual cycle	Periods can become heavier with more pain	Periods become irregular but much lighter. Women often become amenorrhoeic
Menstrual spotting	Often more days of spotting before and after periods	Erratic spotting very common initially but usually settles
Hormonal side effects	None	May cause greasier skin and acne, breast tenderness and mood swings. Symptoms often settle with time
Therapeutic benefits	None	Helps heavy and painful periods. Can use as part of a hormone replacement therapy regimen
Average UK cost	£10	£80

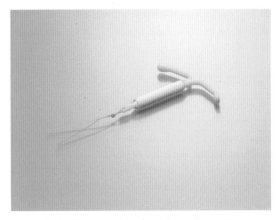

Figure 7.12 Hormone-releasing intrauterine system – Mirena. Photograph courtesy of Bayer Schering Ltd.

Contraindications

There are very few absolute contraindications to the use of intrauterine contraception, but the UKMEC states the following category 4 conditions:

- current STI or PID, including post-abortion and following childbirth;
- malignant trophoblastic disease;
- unexplained vaginal bleeding (before assessment);
- endometrial and cervical cancer (until assessed and treated);
- known malformation of the uterus or distortion of the cavity, for example with fibroids;
- copper allergy (but could use a Mirena).

Special considerations

Infection

The risk of infection with intrauterine contraception has always been overestimated. Although there is a small increase in the risk of pelvic infection in the first few weeks after insertion (just as a consequence of the insertion procedure), it is important to appreciate that the long-term risk is similar to that of women who are not using any method of contraception.

In a mutually monogamous relationship, an IUD user has no increased risk of PID. If an IUD user has a partner with a sexually transmitted infection such as *Chlamydia* or gonorrhoea, the IUD will not protect against these infections, in contrast to condoms or the use of a hormonal method of contraception, which do.

Users of Mirena have a marginally lower overall risk of pelvic infection because of the protective effect of a hormonal method on the upper genital tract.

Antibiotics are not given routinely during insertion of intrauterine contraception but should be considered if a woman is thought to be at higher risk or if there are limited facilities for STI screening.

Ectopic pregnancy

Intrauterine contraception prevents all types of pregnancy, including ectopic pregnancy. However if a pregnancy occurs in a user, the risk of it being ectopic is around 3–5 per cent (<1 per cent for a Mirena). This translates to an overall risk of ectopic pregnancy with a copper IUD of less than 1.5 per 1000 woman-years of IUD use.

Barrier methods of contraception

Barrier methods prevent STIs and are therefore of enormous importance globally. They prevent pregnancy by creating a physical barrier to the sperm reaching and fertilizing the egg. They can be used in conjunction with a hormonal method or IUD to give personal protection against infection and to increase contraceptive efficacy.

Condoms

Male condoms are usually made of latex rubber. They are cheap and are widely available for purchase or free from many clinics. They have been heavily promoted in Safe Sex campaigns to prevent the spread of STIs, particularly HIV.

Condoms of varying sizes and shapes are available and increasingly with different textures, flavours, colours and scents. It is important to use condoms that reach European Union standards and are within their sell-by date. Emergency contraception can be used in the event of a condom bursting or slipping off during intercourse. Some men and women may be allergic to latex condoms or spermicide, and hypoallergenic latex condoms and plastic male condoms are available.

Healthcare professionals may need to teach individuals how to use condoms properly (Figure 7.13). Men must be instructed to apply condoms before any genital contact and to withdraw the erect penis from the vagina immediately after ejaculation.

strongly recommended that individuals at high risk of HIV do not use these products for either vaginal or anal sex.

Female barriers

The diaphragm is the female barrier used most commonly in the UK (Figure 7.14). Various cervical caps are also marketed. They should all be used in conjunction with a spermicidal cream or gel. Diaphragms are inserted immediately prior to intercourse and should be removed no earlier than 6 hours later. Using a diaphragm requires careful teaching and fitting. Female barriers offer protection against pelvic infection, but can increase the risk of urinary tract infection and vaginal irritation.

Female condoms made of plastic are also available (Femidom®). They offer particularly good protection against infection as they cover the whole of the vagina and vulva and, being plastic, are less likely to burst. However, many couples find them unaesthetic and they have not achieved widespread popularity.

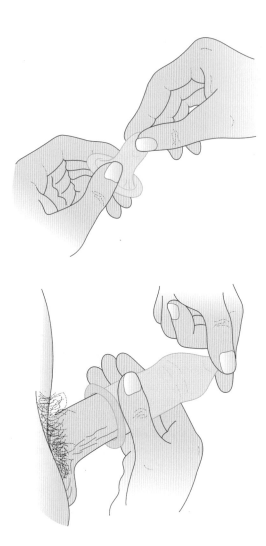

Figure 7.13   Using a condom.

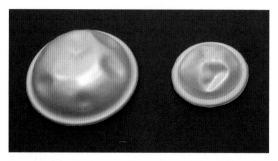

Figure 7.14   Diaphragms. Photograph courtesy of Durbin Ltd.

Spermicides

Very few spermicidal preparations are now available in the UK. The only marketed product is a gel; other countries have a wider range of pessaries, foams and creams. They all contain the active ingredient nonoxynol-9. Spermicides are designed to be used with another barrier method to make them more effective. Nonoxynol-9 may provide protection against some STIs, but a recent concern has been the finding of a higher risk of HIV transmission in frequent spermicide users. For this reason, it is

Withdrawal

Although not strictly speaking a barrier method, withdrawal, or coitus interruptus, is a widespread practice and obviously does not require any medical advice or supplies. The penis is removed from the vagina immediately before ejaculation takes place. Unfortunately, it is not particularly reliable, as pre-ejaculatory secretions may contain millions of sperm and young men often find it hard to judge the timing of withdrawal. The use of emergency contraception should be considered if a couple have used withdrawal (see below).

Natural family planning

This is extremely important worldwide and may be the only type of contraception acceptable to some couples for cultural and religious reasons. It involves abstaining from intercourse during the fertile period of the month.

The fertile period is calculated by various techniques, such as:

- changes in basal body temperature;
- changes in cervical mucus;
- tracking cycle days;
- combined approaches.

Some commercially available kits are available, such as Persona® in the UK, and use readings of urinary hormone levels to define fertile periods when abstinence is required.

The failure rates of natural methods of family planning are quite high, largely because couples find it difficult to abstain from intercourse when required.

The lactational amenorrhoea method (LAM) is used by fully breastfeeding mothers. During the first six months of infant life, full breastfeeding gives more than 98 per cent contraceptive protection.

Emergency contraception

Emergency contraception (EC) is a 'back-up' method that is used after intercourse has taken place and before implantation has occurred. EC should be considered if unprotected intercourse has occurred, if there has been failure of a barrier method, for example a burst condom, or if hormonal contraception has been forgotten.

There are two types of EC in general use:

Hormonal emergency contraception

Levonorgestrel can be taken for EC in a single dose of 1.5 mg (Levonelle®). It has to be used within 72 hours of an episode of unprotected intercourse and the earlier it is taken the more effective it is. There are no real contraindications to its use.

Levonelle® is not 100 per cent effective but will prevent around three-quarters of pregnancies that would otherwise have occurred. It is available free on prescription or over the counter in pharmacies (either to buy or free in some regions). It can be used on more than one occasion in a short space of time, but women should consider other more effective methods if they are using EC repeatedly. The precise mechanism of action is not known, but probably involves disruption of ovulation or corpus luteal function, depending on the time in the cycle when hormonal EC is taken.

A progestogen receptor modulator (ulipristal 30 mg) ellaOne® is now licensed for EC. It is used up to 120 hours following unprotected intercourse or contraceptive failure. It will be available on prescription only in the UK.

An IUD for emergency contraception

A copper IUD can be inserted for EC and is highly effective. It can be inserted up to 5 days after the calculated earliest day of ovulation covering multiple episodes of intercourse in the same menstrual cycle, or up to 5 days after a single episode of unprotected intercourse at any stage in the cycle. The IUD prevents implantation and the copper ions exert an embryo-toxic effect. The normal contraindications to an IUD apply and, if there is a risk of sexually transmitted infection, antibiotic cover should be given. The Mirena has not been shown to be effective for EC and should not be used in this situation.

The copper IUD can remain in situ for ongoing contraception or be removed once the menstrual period has started.

Sterilization

Female sterilization and male vasectomy are permanent methods of contraception and are highly effective. They are usually chosen by relatively older couples who are sure that they have completed their families. Occasionally, individuals who have no children or who, for example, carry an inherited disorder may choose to be sterilized. The uptake of female sterilization and vasectomy in the UK is relatively high compared to many other European countries, with around 50 per cent of couples over the age of 40 years relying on one or other permanent method.

Vasectomy is easier, cheaper and slightly more effective than female sterilization. It does not require a general anaesthetic. Semen analysis has to be checked after the procedure to ensure that it has been successful.

Technically, both female sterilization and vasectomy can be reversed, with subsequent pregnancy rates of about 25 per cent, but reversals are not funded by the NHS in many parts of the UK. Individuals should not have a sterilization procedure performed if there is a chance that one day they might want to have it reversed.

It is estimated that around 10–15 per cent of individuals in the UK subsequently regret the decision to be sterilized. Regret is more common in individuals who are aged less than 30 years at the time, have no children or in women who are within a year of delivery.

Long-acting reversible contraception is highly effective and the option to use these methods instead of a sterilization procedure should always be raised in the counselling session. They are reversible should a woman wish to keep her options open for a future pregnancy.

Consent

It is essential that individuals are very carefully counselled before sterilization and give written consent. Consent forms do not ask for the partner's written consent.

The consent form should clearly indicate that sterilization:

- is a permanent procedure;
- very occasionally can fail.

The failure of sterilization and vasectomy is a major area of medical litigation.

Female sterilization

This involves the mechanical blockage of both Fallopian tubes to prevent sperm reaching and fertilizing the oocyte (Figure 7.15). It can also be achieved by hysterectomy or total removal of both Fallopian tubes.

Female sterilization will not alter the subsequent menstrual pattern as such, but if a woman stops the combined pill to be sterilized, she may find that her subsequent menstrual periods are heavier. Alternatively, if she has an IUD removed at the time of sterilization, she may find her subsequent menstrual periods are lighter.

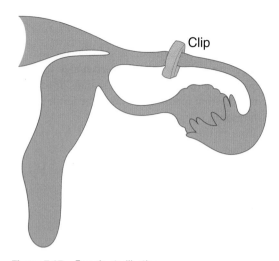

Figure 7.15   Female sterilization.

Sterilization in the UK is most commonly performed by laparoscopy under general anaesthesia, which enables women to be admitted to hospital as a day case. Alternative techniques are mini-laparotomy with a small transverse suprapubic incision or, less commonly, through the posterior vaginal fornix (colpotomy). Mini-laparotomy is the technique of choice when the procedure is carried out post-natally (the uterus is enlarged and more vascular) and in developing countries where laparoscopic equipment is not available. Different ways of occluding the Fallopian tubes are described in Table 7.8.

Essure® is a newer technique which is becoming popular. It involves insertion of metal springs into each Fallopian tube guided by the hysteroscope (Figure 7.16). Scar tissue grows round the metal springs and blocks the tubes. It can be performed under local anaesthetic or light sedation making it a cheaper and easier option than conventional laparoscopic sterilization.

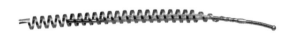

Figure 7.16   Essure sterilization – microinsert. Photograph courtesy of Conceptus Ltd.

Table 7.8   Techniques of female sterilization and their special features

Technique of tubal occlusion	Special features
Clips	Technique of choice in UK
	Several types available
	Occasionally may not occlude whole tube
Fallope rings	Easy to apply
	Damages 2–3 cm of tube, thereby making subsequent reversal more difficult
Ligation	Suitable for postpartum mini-laparotomy
	Has a relatively higher failure rate
Electrocautery/ diathermy	May damage surrounding structures, e.g. bowel and bladder
	Relatively higher late failure rate
Essure	Inserted via hysteroscope under local anaesthetic
	Expanding metal springs placed into Fallopian tubes proximally
Chemical agents, e.g. quinacrine	Inserted via hysteroscope under local anaesthetic
	Not available in the UK, although more widely used in Asia

Complications of female sterilization

Very occasionally, a woman may experience anaesthetic problems or there may be damage to intra-abdominal organs during the procedure. Sometimes it is not possible to visualize the pelvic organs at laparoscopy due to adhesions or obesity; it may then be necessary to proceed to mini-laparotomy.

Female sterilization is highly effective. If it does fail, 30 per cent of pregnancies are likely to be ectopic. Any sterilized woman who misses her period and has symptoms of pregnancy should seek early medical advice.

Vasectomy

Vasectomy involves the division of the vas deferens on each side to prevent the release of sperm during ejaculation (Figure 7.17). It is technically an easier and quicker procedure than female sterilization and is usually performed under local anaesthesia. Various techniques exist to block the vas, and their effectiveness is related primarily to the skill and experience of the operator (Table 7.9).

Vasectomy differs from female sterilization in that it is not effective immediately. Sperm will still be present higher in the genital tract and azoospermia is therefore achieved more quickly if there is frequent

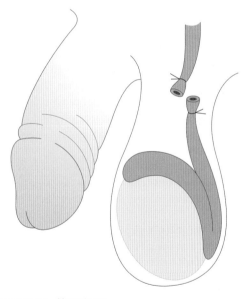

Figure 7.17   Vasectomy.

ejaculation. Men should be advised to hand in two samples of semen at 12 and 16 weeks to see if any sperm are still present. If two consecutive samples are free of sperm, the vasectomy can be considered complete. An alternative form of contraception must be used until that time.

Table 7.9   Techniques of vasectomy

Techniques of vasectomy	Special features
Ligation or clips	Most commonly used
	Unipolar diathermy
Excision	Allows histological confirmation
No-scalpel vasectomy	Widely used in China
	Special instruments used which puncture the skin
	Low incidence of complications
Silicone plugs/ sclerosing agents	Also used in China
	Avoids a skin incision

Complications

Immediate complications such as bleeding, wound infection and haematoma may occur. Occasionally, small lumps may appear at the cut end of the vas as a result of a local inflammatory response. These so-called 'sperm granulomas' may need surgical excision. Some men will develop anti-sperm antibodies following vasectomy. These do not cause symptoms, but if the vasectomy is reversed, pregnancy may not occur because the autoantibodies inactivate sperm. Chronic scrotal pain following a vasectomy is uncommon – one third of men will have pain at 12 weeks post-vasectomy, but only 6–8 per cent of men will still complain of significant discomfort at the end of a year.

Over the years, a possible association between vasectomy and the development of both prostate and testicular cancers has been raised and received widespread media interest. In practice, there is insufficient evidence to support any association.

Abortion

Abortion is one of the most commonly performed gynaecological procedures in the UK. Provision of high quality abortion services with timely access for women is a key sexual health priority. Abortion can be carried out legally up to 24 weeks of gestation.

Women have attempted to end unplanned pregnancies by a variety of methods for centuries. In many countries, illegal abortion still remains the cause of considerable morbidity and mortality. Abortion is a subject that attracts very strong opinions and there is a widespread divergence of views on the subject worldwide, mainly related to cultural and religious backgrounds.

The law and abortion

The UK Abortion Act was passed in 1967. This allows the lawful termination of pregnancies under certain criteria. As a result, illegal abortion in the UK has virtually disappeared. Under the terms of the 1967 Abortion Act, a woman may have an abortion performed if two medical practitioners acting in good faith are willing to certify to one of the following criteria:

- The continuance of the pregnancy would involve risk to the life of the pregnant woman greater than if the pregnancy were terminated.
- The termination is necessary to prevent grave permanent injury to the physical or mental health of the pregnant woman.
- The pregnancy has not exceeded its 24th week and continuance of the pregnancy would involve risk, greater than if the pregnancy were terminated, of injury to the physical or mental health of the pregnant woman.
- The pregnancy has not exceeded its 24th week and continuance of the pregnancy would involve risk, greater than if the pregnancy were terminated, of injury to the physical or mental health of any existing child(ren) of the family of the pregnant woman.
- There is a substantial risk that if the child were born, it would suffer from such physical or mental abnormalities as to be seriously handicapped.
- To save the life of the pregnant woman
- To prevent grave permanent injury to the physical or mental health of the pregnant woman

The form must be signed by both medical practitioners prior to the abortion being performed and posted to the Chief Medical Officer of the Department of Health or of the Scottish Government (Figure 7.18).

IN CONFIDENCE   Certificate A

Not to be destroyed within three
years of the date of the operation

ABORTION ACT 1967
Certificate to be completed in relation to an abortion
under Section 1(1) of the Act

I   ---

(Name and qualifications of practitioner: in Block Capitals)

of   ---

(Full address of practitioner)

Have/have not* seen/examined* the pregnant woman to whom this certificate relates at

*(*delete as appropriate)*

(Full address of place at which patient was seen or examined)

on   ---

and I   ---

(Name and qualifications of practitioner: in Block Capitals)

of   ---

(Full address of practitioner)

Have/have not* seen/and examined* the pregnant woman to whom this certificate relates at

          ----

(Full address of place at which patient was seen or examined)

on   ---

We hereby certify that we are of the opinion formed in good faith, that in the case of

          ----

(Full name of pregnant woman: in Block Capitals)

of   ---

(Usual place of residence of pregnant woman: in Block Capitals)

☐ A the continuance of the pregnancy would involve risk to the life of the pregnant woman
      greater than if the pregnancy were terminated.

☐ B the termination is necessary to prevent grave permanent injury to the physical of mental
      health of the pregnant woman.

Tick appropriate box

☐ C the pregnancy has NOT exceeded its 24th week and that the continuance of the pregnancy
      would involve risk, greater than if the pregnancy were terminated, of injury to the physical or
      mental health of the pregnant woman.

☐ D the pregnancy has NOT exceeded its 24th week and that the continuance of the pregnancy
      would involve risk, greater than if the pregnancy were terminated, of injury to the physical or
      mental health of the existing child(ren) of the family of the pregnant woman.

☐ E there is a substantial risk that if the child were born it would suffer from such physical or mental
      abnormalities as to be seriously handicapped.

This certificate of opinion is given before the commencement of treatment for the termination of pregnancy to which it refers.

Signed --   Date ----------------

Signed --   Date ----------------

Figure 7.18 UK Abortion Act form.

Conscientious objection

Any medical practitioner who has an objection to abortion is not required to participate in abortion services unless the treatment is necessary to save the life of the pregnant woman. However, a medical practitioner who conscientiously objects to abortion should still provide advice and refer a woman promptly to another doctor who would be willing to consider her request sympathetically and arrange the termination if appropriate.

Incidence of legal abortion

Approximately 200 000 abortions are carried out each year in England, Wales and Scotland. Abortion is only permitted in Northern Ireland when it is undertaken to save the life of the pregnant woman. The current abortion rate is around 9–14 per 1000 women aged 15–45 years. This translates to around one in three women having an abortion performed in their lifetime in the UK.

The number of abortions cited for the UK includes women who travel from other countries where abortion is illegal, particularly from the Republic of Ireland. The UK has a significantly lower abortion rate than the USA, but it is still considerably higher than in some western European countries, such as the Netherlands.

Provision of abortion services

In the UK, abortions are carried out within NHS hospitals or in private hospitals and clinics run by charitable organizations depending on the local arrangement. Many NHS regions have set up dedicated abortion services to allow rapid referral and the efficient management of women seeking abortion, staffed by individuals who are particularly sensitive and sympathetic. It is very important that women seeking abortion should not have unnecessary delays in their referral, as increasing gestation increases the risks and complexity of the abortion procedure. Almost all abortions are carried out as day-case procedures.

Assessment and counselling

Prior to an abortion, a woman should have the following assessments.

- Confirmation of the pregnancy by a sensitive pregnancy test.

- Assessment of the gestation: the date of the last menstrual period should be documented. Pelvic and/or abdominal examination is performed. Most women will also have an ultrasound scan.

- Infection screen: all women should be screened for Chlamydia (around one in10 will have a positive result). Consider the need for further STI screening (including HIV and hepatitis B) if the woman has any symptoms (such as abnormal vaginal discharge), is a rape victim or is in a high-risk category. Some units will routinely give antibiotic prophylaxis.

- Haemoglobin and blood grouping: give anti-D immunoglobulin at the time of the procedure if the woman is rhesus negative.

- Cervical smear if this is due.

- Medical history to determine if there is any contraindication to surgery or anaesthetic or a history of allergies or drug reactions.

Pre-abortion counselling is extremely important. The clinician should provide a supportive, non-judgemental setting which offers the woman adequate information and explanation to make an informed choice. Some women will need time to consider their options, while others will be very certain of what they want to do. Consent from the woman's partner is not required. The following areas should be discussed in the counselling process.

- The individual woman's feelings for pregnancy, abortion, her partner, her future life plans and her ability to care for a child at present and in the future.

- The type of abortion that can be performed.

- The risks of the procedure.

- Ensuring the woman has adequate personal support both before and after the abortion.

- Accessing specialist pre- and post-termination support counselling if the decision is particularly difficult.

- Contraception to be used after the abortion.

- Arrangements for follow up.

Abortion techniques

The technique of inducing abortion is determined primarily by gestation. Ideally, an abortion should

Gestation of pregnancy in weeks

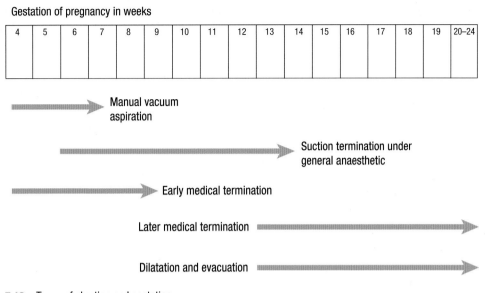

Figure 7.19   Types of abortion and gestation.

always be performed at the earliest possible gestation, as both morbidity and mortality rates rise with increasing gestation. The risk of death from an early surgical termination of pregnancy is less than one per 100 000, which is substantially lower than the maternal mortality associated with a full-term pregnancy.

The discovery of the antiprogestogen mifepristone (or RU 486) has made medical abortion possible. Mifepristone blocks progestogen receptors in the uterus and has been licensed for early abortion since 1991. The licence was subsequently extended to include pregnancies over 13 weeks gestation.

Figure 7.19 shows the options for terminating a pregnancy based on gestation.

First trimester abortion

Surgical

The contents of the uterus are removed by suction using a small plastic cannula inserted through the cervix and attached to an electrical pump or a manual vacuation aspiration (MVA) syringe. Dilatation of the cervix is required to allow a cannula to pass into the uterine cavity, and the greater the gestation of the pregnancy, the greater the amount of dilatation required. Priming of the cervix with agents such as a prostaglandin (inserted into the vagina or taken orally) around 3 hours prior to surgery reduces the risk of cervical trauma and haemorrhage.

Medical

As mifepristone on its own will only induce complete abortion in around 60 per cent of women, it is given in combination with a prostaglandin. This increases the rate of complete abortion to more than 95 per cent. The commonly used schedule is to give 600 mg of oral mifepristone 486, followed 48 hours later by insertion of 1 mg gemeprost vaginal pessary. Lower-dose regimens may be equally effective. Most women stay in hospital for 4–6 hours after insertion of the pessary, during which time most women will abort the pregnancy. The nursing staff confirm passage of the pregnancy. Some UK units facilitate women to remain at home during an early medical abortion.

The medical and surgical methods of early termination are compared in Table 7.10.

Late abortion

Although only about 10–15 per cent of all abortions in the UK are carried out at this stage, mid-trimester abortions are associated with more complications. Major fetal abnormalities detected on ultrasound may necessitate a termination at a very late stage. Not infrequently, the women who present for abortion at advanced gestations are often the very young, or occasionally older women who attribute amenorrhoea to being menopausal.

Table 7.10   Characteristics of early abortion methods

	Surgical	Medical
Effectiveness	Highly	Highly
Average blood loss	Around 80 mL	Around 80 mL
Completeness	95%	95%
Duration	Brief	Takes several days
Anaesthesia	Usually general anaesthesia, but can be done under sedation or local anaesthetic	None
Analgesia	May be required following procedure	Oral or intramuscular analgesia usually required during procedure
Number of visits required	1	2
Availability in the UK	Widespread	Regional variation
Setting	Hospital/clinic	Usually hospital/clinic but can be performed at home
Reason for choice	Unaware of events if general anaesthesia	In control of situation
Patient preference	Equal	Equal
Contraindications	None	Asthma, cardiac disease
Possible complications	Haemorrhage, infection, uterine perforation, cervical damage, failure to remove pregnancy	Haemorrhage, infection, failure to pass products

Medical

Most mid-trimester terminations in the UK involve the pre-treatment administration of mifepristone, followed 36 hours later by vaginal prostaglandin pessaries. A gemeprost pessary is inserted into the vagina every 3–6 hours until the fetus is aborted. Opiate analgesia is usually required, and around 10 per cent of women need a subsequent surgical evacuation of the uterus. The older techniques involving intra-amniotic injections of urea or hypertonic saline combined with intravenous infusions of oxytocin or prostaglandins were relatively inefficient, and it often took women many days to abort. The combination of mifepristone and prostaglandins used currently significantly shortens the time taken to abort the pregnancy to around 6–8 hours.

Surgical

Surgical techniques involve dilatation of the cervix and evacuation of the uterus (D&E) under general anaesthetic. D&E is widely performed in the USA and, although often preferred by women, this procedure is generally disliked by many members of staff as fetal parts may have to be removed piecemeal from the uterus. The procedure should only be performed by specially trained gynaecologists.

Complications of abortion

Incomplete abortion

Placental and/or fetal tissue may remain in the uterus after both medical and surgical abortion. Many women will spontaneously pass the remaining tissue with time, but surgical evacuation of the uterus may be required if there is heavy bleeding or the cervix is still dilated. Very occasionally, the entire pregnancy remains within the uterus after an abortion technique. The woman may then present at an advanced gestation, unaware that the abortion had been unsuccessful.

Infection and subfertility

Pelvic infection following an abortion will present with a febrile illness, an offensive vaginal discharge, lower abdominal pain and tenderness of the pelvic organs on vaginal examination. Antibiotic therapy should be instituted promptly. Infection after an abortion occasionally may cause tubal damage and subsequent subfertility. With modern abortion techniques and screening for pelvic infection, such as *Chlamydia* and gonorrhoea in high-risk women, the risk of subsequent subfertility is very low.

Traumatic injuries

The risk of trauma to the genital tract during an abortion is minimal where there is a high standard of gynaecological practice. During surgical abortion, perforation of the uterus can occur or there may be damage to the cervix, which can predispose to the risk of preterm labour in subsequent pregnancies (cervical incompetence).

Psychological problems

These can be minimized if the woman has been well counselled prior to the abortion. Many women feel emotionally vulnerable in the weeks following an abortion, although for many it is an enormous relief to have the ordeal over. It is quite normal for women to experience feelings of regret and guilt after an abortion, although there is no evidence of an increase in serious psychiatric disease. Many abortion units offer a post-termination support service that women may refer themselves to in the months and even years following an abortion.

Follow up

All women who have had an abortion should be seen for follow up around 2 weeks following the procedure. Most hospitals do not arrange follow-up visits, so this should be carried out in the general practice setting or sexual health clinic. This visit is essential to:

- ensure that the abortion is complete;
- exclude an ongoing pregnancy – the woman should always be examined vaginally;
- check for possible pelvic infection;
- offer advice on contraception and sexual health;
- assess the woman's emotional state.

Contraception

Ovulation may occur within a few weeks of an abortion. It is therefore vital that contraception is discussed prior to the abortion and instituted immediately after the procedure to avoid the chance of a further unplanned pregnancy. Abortion units should provide women with the full range of contraceptive methods.

All hormonal methods should be started on the day of the abortion and Implanon® can be fitted at this stage. An IUD can be inserted at the time of the procedure or, preferably, at the follow-up visit. Barrier methods of contraception can be used immediately. Female sterilization is usually performed 6–8 weeks after an abortion, as it has a higher failure rate when undertaken at the time of surgical abortion.

Hormonal contraception for men

For many decades, scientists have attempted to develop a hormonal method of contraception for men or 'male pill'. Although various agents such as progestogens, antiandrogens and gonadotrophin-releasing hormones all suppress sperm production, they also interfere with sexual function requiring add-back therapy with testosterone. At the present time, there is no licensed male hormonal contraception, although research is continuing.

Key Points

- In the UK, contraception is widely available and is almost always free of charge. Most people use contraception for long periods of time but use different methods at different ages and stages.

- The combined pill is primarily used by young, healthy women and it is estimated that there are around three million current users in the UK.

- Progestogen-only contraception can be used by women with cardiovascular disease and is ideal for breastfeeding or older women.

- Long-acting methods of contraception (LARC) are increasingly recommended as they are highly effective, independent of intercourse and do not rely on any regular activity on the part of the user.

- Condoms should always be recommended in new relationships for personal protection against sexually transmitted infections.

- Natural family planning is an extremely important method worldwide and, for cultural or religious reasons, may be the only method acceptable to some couples.

continued ≫

Key Points *continued*

- Before sterilization, men and women should give written consent to the procedure, which states that they are aware it is permanent and also that it has a very small failure rate.

- Vasectomy is generally an easier, quicker and safer procedure than female sterilization and is usually performed under local anaesthetic.

- Abortion is widely available in the UK. An abortion should be performed at the earliest possible gestation to reduce the risk of complications.

CASE HISTORY

Miss CM is aged 17 years and single. She smokes ten cigarettes a day. She recently became pregnant when a condom burst and has just had an abortion at 14 weeks gestation. Her GP prescribed the combined pill for her in the past, but she thought it made her gain weight and kept forgetting to take it. She has had several partners and now has a new boyfriend. She has no past medical history of note, but was found to be positive for *Chlamydia* when she had her abortion.

As compliance seems to be an important issue here, long-acting methods of contraception should be discussed and can be started immediately. Implanon or Depo-Provera would be options to consider with Miss CM. She would need to be warned about changes in menstrual bleeding patterns with both methods and slight weight gain with Depo-Provera. Intrauterine contraception could be considered but her sexual lifestyle would appear to indicate that she is at higher risk of sexually transmitted infections.

A combined pill could also be prescribed again, with reassurance that weight gain is rarely a significant problem with it. Regular pill taking should be emphasized. Alternatively, the weekly combined hormonal patches could be considered, as she may find compliance easier with them. Spending time with a counselling nurse would be valuable for Miss CM, and back-up leaflets on all the methods would be helpful.

As she is in a new relationship, the use of condoms should be encouraged for personal protection against infection, in combination with a hormonal method. How to use condoms effectively can be demonstrated on a model. If Miss CM decides to use condoms alone, she must be given information about the use and availability of emergency contraception.

Additional reading

Gebbie AE, O'Connell White K. *Fast facts – contraception*, 3rd edn. Oxford: Healthpress Ltd, 2009.

Glasier A, Gebbie A (eds). *The handbook of family planning, and reproductive healthcare*, 5th edn. Edinburgh: Churchill Livingstone, 2007.

Guillebaud J. *Contraception – your questions answered*, 5th edn. Edinburgh: Churchill Livingstone, 2008.

Hatcher RA, Tressell J, Kowal D, Nelson AL. *Contraceptive technology*, 19th edn. New York: Ardent Media Inc., 2007.

Royal College of Obstetricians and Gynaecologists. Male and female sterilisation. Evidence-based clinical guideline no.4. 2004 www.rcog.org.uk/files/rcog-corp/uploaded-files/NEBSterilisationFull060607.pdf.

National Institute for Clinical Excellence (NICE) Long-acting reversible contraception. Clinical guidelines CG30. 2005, www.nice.org.uk/C G030.

Royal College of Obstetricians and Gynaecologists. The care of women requesting induced abortion. Evidence-based clinical guideline no.7. 2004. www.rcog.org.uk/files/rcog-corp/uploaded-files/NEBInducedAbortionfull.pdf.

United Kingdom Medical Eligibility Criteria for Contraceptive use (UKMEC) 2006, www.fsrh.org/admin/uploads/298_UKMEC_200506.pdf.

SUBFERTILITY

OVERVIEW

Subfertility can be primary, in couples who have never conceived, or secondary, in couples who have previously conceived. On average, subfertility affects one in seven couples. It can be defined as failure to conceive after regular sexual intercourse for one or two years in the absence of any known reproductive pathology. The diagnosis of subfertility based on failure to conceive in one year can exaggerate the risk of subfertility as a further 50 per cent of couples will fall pregnant in the subsequent year. Investigations can be justifiably commenced earlier if the couple have a history of predisposing factors such as amenorrhoea, oligomenorrhoea, pelvic inflammatory disease, women with low ovarian reserve or known male factor subfertility. The causes of subfertility can be male, female or mixed. The best model is that of patient-centred care within specialist teams where the patients can be given evidence-based care, adequate counselling and information regarding the relevant support groups.

Natural conception

For a woman with a normal menstrual cycle of 28 days, ovulation occurs around day 14. The average survival time of the oocyte is around 24 hours, while after ejaculation sperm may survive for up to 7 days in the female reproductive tract.

In the general population, up to 90 per cent of couples will have conceived after regular unprotected intercourse for three years (Figure 8.1).

Several general factors may adversely affect the natural conception rate. These are:

- Age: natural conception declines significantly in the female after 35 years of age. This is due to the decline in oocyte quality and numbers.
- Smoking: reduces fertility in females and semen quality in males.
- Coital frequency: stress and anxiety may affect libido and coital frequency and thus impact on fertility. Recommended coital frequency is two to three times per week.
- Alcohol: excessive alcohol is harmful to the fetus, and can also affect sperm quality.
- Body weight: Over or under weight can affect ovulation; women with a body mass index (BMI) of >29 or <19 will have difficulty conceiving.
- Drugs:
  - non-steroidal anti-inflammatory drugs (inhibit ovulation);

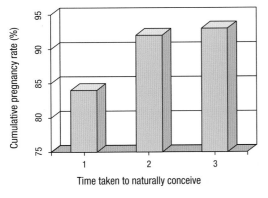

Figure 8.1 The natural conception rate over a three-year period.

- chemotherapy (destroys rapidly dividing cells e.g. gametes);
- cimetidine, sulphasalazine, androgen injections (affects sperm quality).
- Occupational hazards: exposure to chemicals and radiation adversely affects male and female fertility.

Therefore, it is very important to optimize one's health before conception. Besides giving patients life style advice regarding conception, it is also imperative to advise them to take peri-conception folic acid up to 12 weeks gestation as this reduces the risk of neural tube defects; and also offer women rubella screening so that those who are susceptible can be given rubella vaccination to avoid infants being affected with congenital rubella syndrome.

Causes of female subfertility

The main causes of female subfertility can be related to hypothalamic–pituitary–ovarian (HPO) axis dysfunction, ovulatory disorders secondary to ovarian factors, tubal disease and endometrial factors. There is however, also a significant group of patients where their diagnosis is unexplained (Figure 8.2).

Ovulation problems

The landmark physiological process of the development of the human oocyte is illustrated in Figure 8.3. Ovulation is intricately regulated by the HPO axis. Gonadotrophin-releasing hormone (GnRH) controls the release of follicle-stimulating hormone (FSH) and luteinizing hormone (LH) from the pituitary gland, and the process is regulated via a feedback loop. The surge of LH mid-cycle causes ovulation. Where the function of the HPO axis is

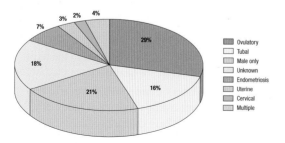

Ovulatory — 29%
Tubal — 16%
Male only — 21%
Unknown — 18%
Endometriosis — 7%
Uterine — 3%
Cervical — 2%
Multiple — 4%

Figure 8.2   Causes of subfertility divided into male and female factors.

disrupted, for example in women with BMI >29 or <19, in polycystic ovarian syndrome (PCOS), hyper- or hypothyroidism and hyperprolactinaemia, ovulation occurs suboptimally.

The most common cause of anovulation is PCOS. Women with PCOS also suffer from menstrual irregularities (usually oligo- or amenorrhoea), increased hair growth (hirsutism), acne and are more commonly overweight. They also are at higher risk of diabetes and cardiovascular disorders. The diagnosis of PCOS is based on a score of two out of three of the Rotterdam criteria (Table 8.1).

Table 8.1   Rotterdam criteria for diagnosis of PCOS

Revised 2003 criteria (2 out of 3 for diagnosis)
1. Oligo- or anovulation
2. Clinical and/or biochemical signs of hyperandrogenism
3. Polycystic ovaries on ultrasound and exclusion of other aetiologies (congenital adrenal hyperplasia, androgen-secreting tumors, Cushing syndrome)

Marker of ovarian reserve

In the ovary, anti-Müllerian hormone (AMH) is produced by the granulosa cells. AMH levels can be measured in blood and are shown to be proportional to the number of small antral follicles. In women, serum AMH levels decrease with age and are undetectable in the post-menopausal period. AMH levels represent the quantity of the ovarian follicle pool and are a useful marker of ovarian reserve. AMH measurement can also be useful in the prediction of the extremes of ovarian response to gonadotrophin stimulation for *in vitro* fertilization, namely poor and hyper-response.

Tubal blockage

Tubal blockage can be the result of previous pelvic inflammatory disease, such as a *Chlamydia* infection, but can also be the result of any inflammatory process within the abdominal/pelvic cavity. Inflammatory processes as a result of surgery or endometriosis may result in the formation of internal scars, called adhesions, which may result in organs adhering abnormally to each other. If the Fallopian tubes are involved, then this may result in partial or complete blockage of the tubes (Figure 8.4).

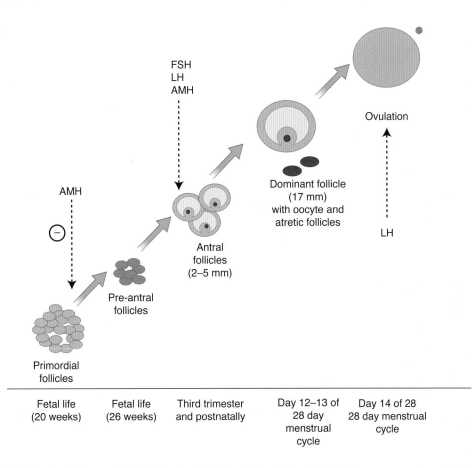

Figure 8.3 Landmark stages of follicular development during fetal and later life. In the human ovary, primordial follicles are present by 20 weeks. By 26 weeks, pre-antral follicles (primary and secondary) are formed. AMH inhibits the transition from the primordial to the primary follicular stage. AMH is also important in the regulation of FSH induced oocyte growth and the cyclic selection of the dominant follicle. AMH, anti-Mullerian hormone; FSH, follicular stimulating hormones; LH, luteinizing hormone.

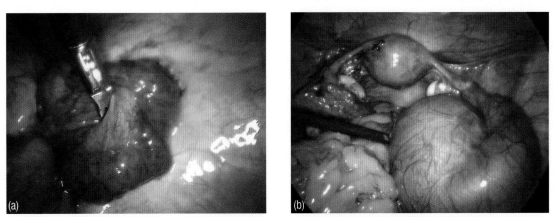

Figure 8.4 (a) Photograph of a normal fimbrae end of a Fallopian tube during laparoscopy. (b) Photograph of a right hydrosalpinx.

Endometrial factors

Abnormalities within the endometrium may prevent the successful implantation of the embryo. The endometrium or the cavity may be abnormal in the presence of uterine fibroids (Figure 8.5), adhesions and polyps. These pathologies can often be surgically managed to improve the chances of conception.

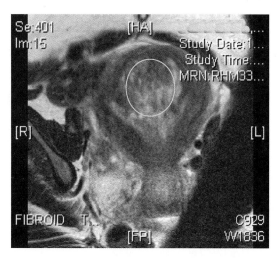

Figure 8.5 Magnetic resonance image of a large fibroid within the cavity of the uterus (yellow circle).

Causes of male subfertility

In the human, the process of spermatogenesis starts at puberty and continues throughout life. The total process of spermatogenesis in humans takes 74 days within the seminiferous tubules. It takes a further ten days for the sperm to travel to the epididymis to be stored for use during ejaculation. The head of the epididymis stores 70 per cent of the mature sperm and, during ejaculation, the sperm exit via the vas deferens which then passes through the inguinal canal and opens into the urethra adjacent to the prostate.

The supporting cells of the testis are the Leydig and Sertoli cells. The Leydig cells are contained in the connective tissue of the testis and are the prime source of the male hormone, testosterone. LH from the pituitary gland regulates Leydig cell function by the negative feedback loop. The Sertoli cells are highly specialized cells that maintain the integrity of the seminiferous epithelium (so that spermatogenesis can occur in an immune privileged area) as well as nourish the developing sperm.

Approximately one in 20 men are subfertile, about 85 per cent have suboptimal semen quality, while azoospermia, coital dysfunction and immune factors contribute to the rest. The causes for male subfertility are listed in Figure 8.6. Any factors, whether genetic, physiological, pathological or mechanical, that affect the spermatogenesis process from the production to time of ejaculation will influence male fertility.

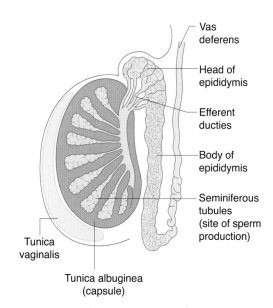

Figure 8.6 Illustration of the anatomy of the testis and the possible causes of male subfertility.

History and examination

Table 8.2 illustrates the key points in performing history and examination in patients with subfertility.

Table 8.2   Key points to cover in history and examination of patients presenting with subfertility

History	
Female	**Male**
Length of time spent trying for pregnancy	Length of time spent trying for pregnancy
Any previous pregnancies	Fathered any previous pregnancies
Coital frequency	History of mumps or measles
Occupation	History of testicular trauma, surgery to testis
Menstrual history	Occupation
Previous history of pelvic inflammatory disease	Medical and surgical history
Previous medical and surgical history	
Previous fertility treatment	
Cervical smear history	
General health – screen for history of thyroid disorders	
Examination	
Pelvic examination – any uterine pathology such as fibroids	Testicular examination – testicular volume, consistency, masses, absence of vas deferens, varicocele, evidence of surgical scars
General BP, pulse, height and weight	

Investigations

Investigations are necessary to check for HPO dysfunction (follicular phase FSH, LH, oestradiol), tubal patency (hysterosalpingogram (HSG), hysterocontrast synography (HyCoSy) or an operative laparoscopy and dye test) and semen analysis for males. In general, tubal patency is checked using either HSG or HyCoSy as screening tests, and if these tests suggest potential blockage of the Fallopian tubes, then the patient can be counselled regarding the need to undergo an operative laparoscopy and dye test for diagnostic purposes; with the intention of treating any pelvic pathology that can be surgically corrected at the time of operation.

HSG and HyCoSy are both comparable in terms of effectiveness as screening tests for tubal patency. Both require instrumentation of the uterine cavity and instilling radio-opaque dye (HSG) or sono-opaque contrast medium (HyCoSy) via a very fine catheter (Figure 8.7). During HSG, the time lapse of the flow of dye is captured by x-rays while in HyCoSy, it is visualized via an ultrasound scan. If there is a blockage of the Fallopian tube, dye will be seen to accumulate in a pocket representing the blocked end of the Fallopian tube (Figure 8.7).

It is crucial that one remembers that tubal patency is not equivalent to tubal function. Currently, there is as yet no effective test to check for tubal function.

Semen analysis

Semen analysis should be performed after the patients have abstained from sexual intercourse for 3–4 days. Two abnormal test results are required to diagnose male subfertility. The normal sperm parameters are shown in Table 8.3.

For men with a very low sperm count or azoospermia, it is important to check their testosterone levels (low levels suggest a production impairment) and LH/FSH. (Hypogonadotrophic hypogonadism is rare and can be treated with FSH and hCG injections.) It is also important to screen for the cystic fibrosis (CF) mutation as a congenital bilateral absence of the vas deferens (CBAVD) is a minor variant of cystic fibrosis. If the male partner

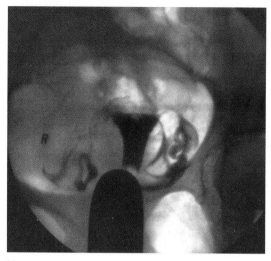

(a)

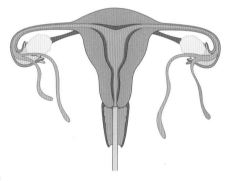

(b)

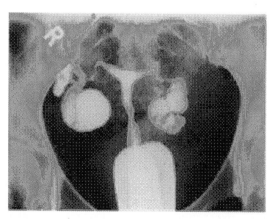

(c)

Figure 8.7 (a) Hysterosalpingogram (HSG) showing normal patency of the fallopian tubes; (b) Pictorial illustration of a normal HSG. (c) Abnormal HSG with pocketed areas suggesting blocked tubes.

Table 8.3 Normal parameters for semen analysis (WHO criteria)

Volume	>2 mL
pH	>7.2
Sperm concentration	>20 million per mL
Total sperm number	>40 million per ejaculate
Motility	>50% grade a and b
Morphology	>30% normal forms

is found to have the CF mutation, it is important to screen the female partner for it. If both partners are carriers, there is a one in four chance of the child being affected by CF and therefore the couple will require pre-conceptual genetic counselling prior to assisted conception. Karyotyping is also offered as there may be Y chromosome deletion defects (AZF region). Specific types of Y chromosome deletion, namely AZFa and AZFb Y chromosome deletions, carry poor prognosis for surgical sperm retrieval procedures.

Management of subfertility

Medical and surgical management are complementary to each other and fertility treatment must be individualized to optimize the treatment result (Table 8.4).

Ovulation induction

The most common anti-oestrogen agent used is clomifene citrate (CC). CC induce gonadotrophin release by occupying the oestrogen receptors in the hypothalamus, thereby interfering with the normal feedback mechanisms, increasing the release of FSH and so stimulating the ovary to produce more follicles. Approximately 70 per cent of women on CC will ovulate, with a pregnancy rate of 15–20 per cent. There is a risk of multiple pregnancies (10 per cent) and therefore women on CC should be monitored by ultrasound scans to track the growth of their follicles.

Ovulation induction (OI) can also be induced by laparoscopic ovarian drilling (LOD). For unknown reasons, passing electrical energy through polycystic ovaries can result in the induction of ovulation. However, as LOD is a surgical procedure with the attached risks associated with surgery and

Table 8.4 Summary of the medical and surgical management of subfertility

Medical	Treatment criteria
Ovulation induction (OI) – clomifene or FSH	Anovulation – PCOS, idiopathic
Intrauterine insemination (IUI) – with or without stimulation with FSH	Unexplained subfertility
Anovulation unresponsive to OI	
Mild male factor	
Minimal to mild endometriosis	
Donor insemination (DI) – with or without stimulation with FSH	Presence of azospermia
Single women	
Same sex couples	
In vitro fertilization (IVF)	Patients with tubal pathology
Patients who underwent above treatment with no success in pregnancy	
Donor egg with IVF	Women whose egg quality is poor, e.g. older women, premature ovarian failure
Previous surgery/chemo-radiotherapy where ovarian function was adversely affected	
Surgical	**Treatment criteria**
Operative laparoscopy to treat disease and restore anatomy	Adhesions
Endometriosis	
Ovarian cyst	
Myomectomy – hysteroscopy, laparoscopy, laparotomy, fibroid embolization	Fibroid uterus
Tubal surgery	Blocked Fallopian tubes amenable to repair
Laparoscopic ovarian drilling	PCOS unresponsive to medical treatment

anaesthesia, it is only appropriate to offer such treatment to women who have not responded to CC treatment.

OI can also be performed by offering a small dose of FSH to induce follicular growth. The process will require follicular tracking with ultrasound scans to minimize the risk of multifollicular ovulation and the risk of multiple pregnancies.

Intrauterine insemination (IUI)

Intrauterine insemination (IUI) is performed by introducing a small sample of prepared sperm into the uterine cavity with a fine uterine catheter. This process usually requires mild stimulation with FSH to produce 2–3 mature follicles. Follicular tracking is essential to avoid over or under stimulation. The success rate of this procedure ranges between 15 and 20 per cent in top fertility units.

In vitro fertilization

Figure 8.8 illustrates a typical *in vitro* fertilization (IVF) treatment cycle. The success rate of IVF per cycle is about 30 per cent in women under 35 years of age. In essence, the ovaries are stimulated with

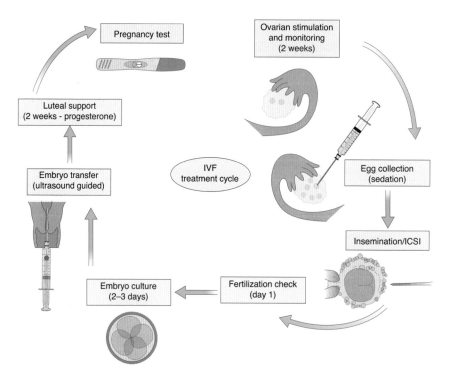

Figure 8.8 An IVF treatment cycle.

FSH, and are encouraged to produce up to 8–10 follicles. Induction of ovulation is then performed with an injection of hCG, after which the eggs can be collected during an ultrasound guided procedure via a very fine needle. These eggs will be fertilized in a petri dish with sperm or, if required, the sperm can be injected directly into the egg (intracytoplasmic sperm injection, ICSI). When fertilization occurs, the fertilized embryo(s) is then replaced into the uterine cavity. Approximately 2 weeks after embryo transfer, a pregnancy test is performed to check for successful implantation.

Undergoing IVF does not preclude the patient from the normal complications of pregnancy, such as miscarriage or ectopic pregnancies. The risk of ectopic pregnancy for women who have undergone IVF is higher than for the general population, at 3–4 per cent. There is the added risk of overstimulating the ovaries during an IVF cycle. Patients with ovarian hyperstimulation syndrome (OHSS) present with ascites, hugely enlarged multifollicular ovaries, pulmonary oedema, and are at risk of multiorgan failure and coagulopathy. These patients need to be admitted to hospital and managed under strict protocols under the care of specialist teams.

Surgical sperm retrieval

Where the sperm quality is low but sperm are present, ICSI is required to help achieve a pregnancy. However, in the absence of naturally ejaculated sperm, patients will have to undergo surgical sperm retrieval (SSR). SSR can be performed under sedation or general anaesthetic. A fine needle is inserted into the epididymis or the testicular tissue to obtain sperm or testicular tissue with sperm, respectively. The retrieved sperm can then be cryopreserved or injected into the oocyte as part of a fresh IVF/ICSI cycle.

Cryopreservation of gametes

Sperm or oocyte can be cryopreserved for later use. Often this process is very useful in preserving fertility for patients undergoing chemo/radiation therapy for cancer. Currently, the pregnancy rate for thawed sperm/egg in top fertility centres is very near to that of normal IVF cycles. This process can also be used for storage of gametes from donors who wish to donate their sperm or eggs for altruistic reasons to help couples with fertility problems.

Key Points

- In the assessment of subfertility a careful history, examination, investigation and, when necessary, counselling should include both partners

- The couple should be given information on the natural conception rate (including the impact of advancing age), advice on life style issues relating to diet, smoking, weight and alcohol consumption so that they can optimize their peri-conception health

- Ovarian reserve decreases significantly after the age of 35 years

- Fertility treatment is a combination of surgical and medical treatments which are complementary to each other

- A step-wise strategy of assisted conception includes: (1) ovulation induction; (2) intrauterine insemination and (3) IVF/ICSI.

- The investigations of male subfertility include karyotyping, screening for CF (CBAVD), testosterone, FSH and LH concentrations

- Male partners with azospermia can undergo SSR to retrieve sperm

- Sperm and eggs can be electively cryopreserved in certain clinical circumstances, such as prior to chemo/radiotherapy.

CHAPTER 9

PROBLEMS IN EARLY PREGNANCY

OVERVIEW

The two large groups of early pregnancy problems are ectopic pregnancy and miscarriage. Both these conditions can be life threatening and are commonly seen in our gynaecology emergency department. Other early pregnancy problems that are less common include (Table 9.1) gestational trophoblastic disorder, urinary tract infection, hyperemesis gravidarum and medical/surgical problems.

Ectopic pregnancy

Definition

Ectopic pregnancy is defined as implantation of a conceptus outside the normal uterine cavity.

Incidence and aetiology

The incidence of ectopic pregnancy in the UK is 11/1000 pregnancies and the mortality rate is around 10/100 000. Approximately 11 000 cases of ectopic pregnancies are diagnosed each year in the UK. The rising incidence of ectopic pregnancy can in some way be related to the fact that early diagnosis of pregnancy can be made with the use of β-human chorionic gonadotrophin (βHCG) and ultrasound scans to identify the location of an early pregnancy.

Heterotopic pregnancy is the simultaneous development of a pregnancy within and outside the uterine cavity. Although the incidence of a heterotopic pregnancy in the general population is low (1:25 000– 30 000), the incidence is significantly higher after *in vitro* fertilization (IVF) treatment (1 per cent).

Common sites of implantation within the abdominal cavity are the Fallopian tubes (95 per cent), ovaries (3 per cent) and peritoneal cavity (1 per cent). In the Fallopian tubes, the distribution of sites of implantation are the ampulla (74 per cent), isthmus (12 per cent), fimbrial end of the tube (12 per cent) and interstitium (2 per cent).

Known aetiological factors contributing to the risk of ectopic pregnancy are:

- tubal disease; pelvic infection, such as *Chlamydia* infection, has been estimated to account for 40 per cent of all ectopic pregnancies;
- previous ectopic pregnancy;
- previous tubal surgery;
- subfertility;
- use of intrauterine device.

Clinical presentation

The majority of patients present with a subacute clinical picture of abdominal pain and vaginal bleeding in early pregnancy. Vaginal bleeding is usually dark red, indicative of old blood. The abdominal/pelvic pain may be localized to the iliac fossa. Occasionally, patients have shoulder tip pain indicative of free blood in the abdominal cavity causing diaphragmatic irritation and symptoms of dizziness (anaemia).

Bimanual examination can reveal tenderness in the fornices and there may be cervical excitation, again suggesting peritoneal irritation by free blood.

However, some patients can present very acutely with rupture of the ectopic pregnancy and massive intraperitoneal bleeding. They can present with signs of hypovolaemic shock and acute abdomen.

Table 9.1   Summary of the clinical presentation, epidemiology, risk factors and management of several other early pregnancy disorders not discussed in detail in this chapter

Disorder	Epidemiology	Risk factors	Clinical presentation	Management
Gestational trophoblastic disorder (GTD)	Complete mole: 1/1000 Partial mole: 1/700 (Disorder of the placenta trophoblast)	Previous molar pregnancy, high maternal age, ABO blood group	Persistent elevated βHCG levels after pregnancy/ miscarriage Ultrasound features 'snow storm' appearance	Uterine evacuation followed by βHCG follow up
Urinary tract infection (UTI)	6% of pregnant women have asymptomatic bacteruria. These have a 30% chance of developing a UTI in pregnancy	Pregnancy, previous UTIs, history of renal disorders	Pyrexia, unwell, dysuria, haematuria	Antibiotics Radiological investigations, such as renal scans, may be required
Hyperemesis gravidarum	Occurs in about 1–2% of pregnancies	Non-Caucasian population, multiple gestation, GTD	Severe and intractable vomiting in pregnancy, abdominal pain	Fluid and electrolyte replacement Ultrasound scan Antiemetics and multivitamin replacement

Investigation

The following are useful investigations for the diagnosis of ectopic pregnancy.

- Observations: BP, pulse, temperature
- Laboratory investigations: Haemoglobin, group and save (or crossmatch if patient is severely compromised) and βHCG.
- HCG: This hormone is a glycoprotein produced by the placenta. It has a half-life of up to 24 hours and peaks at around ten weeks. Pregnancy tests measure the β-subunit of HCG. A βHCG level of less than 5 mIU/mL is considered negative for pregnancy, and anything above 25 mIU/mL is considered positive for pregnancy. In 85 per cent of pregnancies, the βHCG levels almost double every 48 hours in a normally developing pregnancy. In patients with ectopic pregnancies, the rise of βHCG is often suboptimal. However,

βHCG levels can vary widely in individuals and thus often multiple readings are required for comparison purposes.

- Transvaginal ultrasound scan (TVS): An intrauterine gestational sac should be visualized at about 4.5 weeks of gestation. The corresponding βHCG at that gestation is around 1500 mIU/mL. By the time a gestational sac with fetal heart pulsation is detected (at around 5 weeks gestation), βHCG level should be around 3000 mIU/mL. Hence, the interpretation of βHCG must be done in context with the clinical picture and ultrasound findings. Thus, if there were discrepancy between the βHCG concentrations and that seen on ultrasound scan (e.g. a high βHCG with no intrauterine pregnancy on ultrasound scan), the differential diagnosis of an ectopic pregnancy must be made. Identification of an intrauterine pregnancy (gestation sac, yolk sac along with fetal pole) on TVS effectively excludes the possibility of an ectopic pregnancy in most patients except in those patients with rare heterotopic pregnancy. The presence of free fluid during TVS is suggestive of a ruptured ectopic pregnancy.

- Laparoscopy: this can be used to diagnose and treat ectopic pregnancy.

Management

Ectopic pregnancy can be managed using an expectant, medical or a surgical approach, depending on clinical presentation and patient choice.

Expectant

Expectant management is based on the assumption that a significant proportion of all tubal pregnancies will resolve through regression or a tubal abortion without any treatment. This option is suitable for patients who are haemodynamically stable and asymptomatic. This entails serial βHCG measurements and ultrasonography.

Medical

Systemic methotrexate is a treatment option for a carefully selected subgroup of patients. Methotrexate, a folic acid antagonist, inhibits DNA synthesis in trophoblastic cells. It can be administered as a single intramuscular injection or in a multiple fixed dose regimen. The dose is calculated based on the patient's body surface area and is 50 mg/m^2.

The following are reasonable indications for the use of methotrexate: (1) cornual pregnancy; (2) persistent trophoblastic disease; (3) patient with one Fallopian tube and fertility desired; (4) patient who refuses surgery or in whom risks of surgery is too high; and (5) treatment of ectopic pregnancy where trophoblast is adherent to bowel or blood vessel. Medical treatment should be offered only if facilities are present for regular follow-up visits.

The few contraindications to medical treatment include (1) chronic liver, renal or haematological disorder; (2) active infection; (3) immunodeficiency; and (4) breastfeeding. There are also known side effects such as nausea, vomiting, stomatitis, conjunctivitis, gastrointestinal upset, photosensitive skin reaction and about two-thirds of patients suffer nonspecific abdominal pain. It is important to advise women to avoid sexual intercourse during treatment and to take some form of contraception for three months after methotrexate treatment. It is also important to avoid alcohol and exposure to sunlight during treatment.

Surgical management

Surgical treatment can be by laparoscopy or laparotomy. The laparoscopic approach offers significant advantage when compared to laparotomy as it results in less blood loss, shorter operating time, less analgesia requirement, a shorter hospital stay and a shorter convalescence than laparotomy. Laparoscopic surgery is the mainstay of management. Laparotomy is mainly reserved for severely compromised patients or due to the lack of endoscopic facilities.

During surgery, the Fallopian tube can either be removed (salpingectomy) or a small opening can be made at the site of the ectopic pregnancy and the trophoblastic tissue extracted via the opening (salpingotomy). In general, if the patient has a normal remaining tube, salpingectomy is the treatment of choice. Salpingotomy is thought to be associated with a higher rate of subsequent ectopic pregnancy.

Key Points

- Management of an ectopic pregnancy should be based on the clinical presentation, βHCG and ultrasound findings

- An intrauterine gestational sac should be visualized at about 4.5 weeks of gestation via TVS, with the corresponding βHCG at that gestation being around 1500 mIU/mL.

- Identification of an intrauterine pregnancy (gestation sac, yolk sac along with fetal pole) on TVS effectively excludes the possibility of an ectopic pregnancy in most patients, except in those with rare heterotopic pregnancy.

- Methotrexate is an option for a selected group of patients who are haemodynamically stable and compliant. Units offering this treatment must be well equipped to deal with out-of-hour emergencies and must be able to offer follow-up visits.

- Surgical treatment will remain the mainstay treatment modality for ectopic pregnancy in most units.

Miscarriage

Miscarriage is a pregnancy that ends spontaneously before the fetus has reached a viable gestational age. At present, the legal definition of miscarriage in the UK is spontaneous loss of pregnancy at or before 24 weeks gestation.

Risk of miscarriage

Sporadic miscarriage is the most common complication of pregnancy. The incidence in a clinical recognizable pregnancy is 10–20 per cent. The incidence decreases after the 8th week of pregnancy to about 10 per cent, with the risk decreased to 3 per cent if a viable fetus has been recognized on ultrasound scan. Maternal age is an independent risk factor for miscarriage. Advanced maternal age leads to a decreased number of good quality oocytes and an increased risk of miscarriage.

Several other uncommon factors that can contribute to early pregnancy losses are:

- chromosomal abnormalities;
- medical/endocrine disorders;
- uterine abnormalities;
- infections;
- drugs/chemicals.

Types of miscarriage

Clinically, miscarriages can be classified into different types based on the clinical presentation and investigation findings. Table 9.2 illustrates the respective clinical presentation, and the examination findings of the respective types of miscarriages.

Management

On initial assessment, a history and examination should be performed with the following:

- observations: BP, pulse, temperature;
- laboratory investigations: haemoglobin, group and save (or crossmatch if patient is severely compromised);
- patients with miscarriage can have expectant, medical or surgical management.

Expectant

The natural course of early pregnancy loss is unknown, and it is questionable if all women with a miscarriage should have any intervention at all. Expectant management allows for the avoidance of surgery and general anaesthesia; patients also potentially feel more in control. Women undergoing expectant care may require unplanned surgery if they start to bleed heavily.

Surgical

Surgical management or evacuation of products of conception (ERPC) has a high success rate of 95–100 per cent. However, surgical evacuation has its drawbacks including risks such as cervical trauma and subsequent cervical incompetence, uterine

Table 9.2   Types of miscarriages with the relevant ultrasound findings and clinical presentation

Type of miscarriage	Ultrasound findings	Clinical presentation
Threatened miscarriage	Intrauterine pregnancy	Per vaginal bleeding and pain Speculum: cervical os close
Inevitable miscarriage	Intrauterine pregnancy	Per vaginal bleeding and pain Speculum: cervical os open
Incomplete miscarriage	Retained products of conception	Per vaginal bleeding and pain Speculum: cervical os open, products of conception located in cervical os
Complete miscarriage	No retained products of conception	Pain and bleeding has resolved Speculum: cervical os closed
Missed miscarriage	Fetal pole present, but no fetal heartbeat identified Gestational sac present (diameter >20 mm) but no fetal pole identified	With or without pain and bleeding

perforation, intrauterine adhesions or postoperative pelvic infection. The incidence of serious morbidity is about 2 per cent with a mortality of 0.5/100 000. Very occasionally, moderate to severe adhesions can result from ERPC and these adhesions can result in subfertility and can be a challenge to treat.

Medical management

About 20 per cent of women with miscarriage will opt for medical management. Prostaglandins are used in single or divided doses administered orally (misoprostol) or vaginally (Gemeprost). Misoprostol is cheap and effective in both oral and vaginal forms. Often, mifepristone (a progesterone antagonist) is used together with prostaglandins to increase the success rate of medical management. Again, women undergoing medical management of miscarriage need to understand that they may need surgical treatment if medical treatment fails.

Counselling services

Patients who have suffered miscarriages should be offered counselling to ensure that they understand that most miscarriages are nonrecurrent. They should also be provided with the necessary psychological support where necessary.

Key Points

- Miscarriages occur in 20 per cent of pregnant women and are mostly due to nonrecurrent cause.
- Advanced maternal age is one of the key factors for miscarriages.
- Women presenting with possible miscarriage should have a clinical history, examination and arranged to have a TVS, where needed. βHCG may occasionally be necessary when the pregnancy site is unknown.
- Patients can be offered the options of expectant, medical and surgical management, depending on clinical presentation and patient choice.
- Patients should also be supported with adequate counselling services.

CASE HISTORY

Mrs AB was admitted to the gynaecological emergency with moderate abdominal pain. She is known to be around 6 weeks pregnant. She gives a 2-day history of vaginal bleeding of dark coloured blood, and presented with newly onset shoulder tip pain and dizziness. Her observations on admission were BP 100/50 mmHg, pulse 100/min, temperature 36.9°C.

Ultrasound scan revealed an adnexa mass on the right and some free fluid in the pelvis. There was no gestational sac in the uterus. βHCG sent by her GP a day ago was 4000 IU/L.

What is your differential diagnosis?

Ectopic pregnancy.

Discuss management

The patient had a large bore cannula inserted and was given i.v. fluids. Bloods were taken for full blood count and group and save. Discussions were made with senior colleagues about her admission and possibility of requiring a laparoscopy.

The patient had a laparoscopy and was discovered to have a large right ectopic pregnancy in her Fallopian tube. She had a salpingectomy and subsequently recovered well.

Additional reading

Dempsey A. Early pregnancy disorders: An update and eye to the future. *Semin Reprod Med* 2008; **26**: 401–10.

Garry R. Laparoscopic surgery. *Best Pract Res Clin Obstet Gynaecol* 2006; **20**: 89–104.

Hinshaw K, Cooper K, Henshaw R *et al.* Management of uncomplicated miscarriage. *BMJ* 1993; **307**: 259.

Royal College of Obstetricians and Gynaecologists. *The management of tubal pregnancy.* Green top guideline no 21. London: RCR/RCOG, May 2004.

Royal College of Obstetricians and Gynaecologists. *The Management of early pregnancy loss.* Green top guideline. London: RCR/RCOG, October 2006.

CHAPTER 10

BENIGN DISEASES OF THE UTERUS AND CERVIX

OVERVIEW

Benign diseases of the cervix and body of the uterus are common problems presenting in almost every gynaecological outpatient clinic. The most common myometrial problem is uterine fibroids. Adenomyosis and endometriosis is dealt with in Chapter 11, Endometriosis and adenomyosis.

Benign diseases of the uterus may be classified in terms of the tissue of origin: the uterine cervix, the endometrium and the myometrium.

The uterine cervix

The cervix is an integral part of the uterus, made up of collagen fibres. It is lined by non-keratinized stratified squamous epithelium in the vaginal part (ectocervix), which changes into columnar epithelium in the endocervical canal. There is a clear demarcation of this transformation between the two types of epithelium, called the 'squamocolumnar junction'. This anatomical junction fluctuates with hormonal influence.

Cervical ectropion

This is a benign condition which looks like a 'raw' area on the cervix. This is due to the presence of columnar epithelium found on the vaginal aspect of the cervix. It can present with an excessive clear odourless mucus-type discharge. A cervical ectropion is commonly and erroneously named 'cervical erosion'. An ectropion commonly develops under the influence of the three Ps: puberty, pill and pregnancy. If the discharge becomes troublesome, the predisposing factor can be stopped or the cervix ablated if the cervical cytology is normal. An infection screen to exclude *Chlamydia* and other sexually transmitted infections should be performed prior to treatment. A persistent cervical ectropion (being a 'weaker' columnar epithelium)

undergoes metaplasia to a 'stronger' squamous epithelium. This transformation zone undergoes dyskaryosis and possible malignant change due to HPV infection, which is subject to screening by cervical cytology. Sometimes the columnar glands within the transformation zone become sealed over, forming small (2–10 mm), mucus-filled cysts visible on the ectocervix. These are termed 'Nabothian follicles' and are of no pathological significance. No treatment is usually required.

Cervical stenosis

Cervical stenosis is usually an iatrogenic phenomena caused by a surgical event. Treatment of pre-malignant disease of the cervix using cone biopsy or loop diathermy can cause cervical stenosis. The recent increased use of endometrial ablation devices has seen a higher incidence of cervical stenosis, particularly where the internal cervical os (isthmus) has been ablated. The ensuing haematometra (blood collected within uterus which is unable to be released through the cervix) causes cyclical dysmenorrhoea with no associated menstrual bleeding. Treatment is by surgical dilatation of the cervix with hysteroscopic guidance, which can be carried out under local anaesthesia. Re-stenosis can occur and sometimes hysterectomy is required to relieve the pain.

Endometrium

The uterine endometrium comprises glands and stroma with a complex architecture, including blood vessels and nerves. During the follicular phase of the menstrual cycle, proliferation of tissue from the basal layer occurs under the predominant influence of oestrogen. After ovulation, the secretory phase change is primarily under the influence of progesterone. In a regular cycle, the secretory phase is a constant 14 days. Menstruation occurs with endometrial shedding as progesterone levels fall.

Disorders of the endometrium give rise to abnormal uterine bleeding (Chapter 5, Disorders of the menstrual cycle). Within this umbrella sit conditions such as post-menopausal bleeding (PMB), intermenstrual bleeding (IMB) and heavy menstrual bleeding (HMB), including bleeding of endometrial origin (BEO) (Chapter 5, Disorders of the menstrual cycle).

Endometrial polyps

Endometrial polyps are discrete outgrowths of endometrium, attached by a pedicle, which move with the flow of the distension medium. They may be pedunculated or sessile, single or multiple and vary in size (0.5–4 cm). In women under 40 years of age, endometrial polyps are unlikely to be of any significance. They may cause intermenstrual bleeding, but only require treatment by removal if the symptom is persistent for at least three months or more.

In women over the age of 40 and pre-menopausal, endometrial polyps diagnosed by ultrasound or hysteroscopy should be considered for removal. In most cases, this can now be carried out in the outpatient setting under local anaesthesia. With increasing age, the most common abnormality is endometrial hyperplasia, which can be present in just the endometrial polyp tissue. Removal of the polyp usually resolves the patient symptoms.

Post-menopausally, it is mandatory to remove endometrial polyps which can be due to hyperplasia or malignancy. Polyps can also be caused by tamoxifen treatment for breast cancer and can be present in up to 30 per cent of such cases. In most cases, the polyps are benign but removal is necessary to exclude the remote possibility of malignancy.

Asherman syndrome

Irreversible damage of the single layer thick basal endometrium does not allow normal regeneration of the endometrium. The endometrial cavity undergoes fibrosis and adhesion formation, termed 'Asherman syndrome'. The result is reduced, or absent, menstrual shedding. This can occur with overzealous curettage of the uterine cavity during evacuation of retained products of conception after miscarriage or following secondary postpartum haemorrhage. In this 'soft' uterine state, the myometrium (including the basal layer) can be inadvertently excavated, causing the problem. Similarly, the same principle is deliberately intended following endometrial destruction, a surgical treatment for menorrhagia where a diathermy loop or ball (first generation) and ablative methods (second generation devices such as hot water balloon, bipolar diathermy, laser or microwave) are used to destroy the basal layer. As Asherman syndrome is difficult to treat in most cases, the mainstay of treatment is preventative. Current treatment options involve hysteroscopic techniques to manually break down or lyse the intrauterine adhesions. Other causes of Asherman syndrome are tuberculosis and schistosomiasis.

Myometrium: uterine fibroids

Pathology

A fibroid is a benign tumour of uterine smooth muscle, termed a 'leiomyoma'. The gross appearance is of a firm, whorled tumour located adjacent to and bulging into the endometrial cavity (submucous fibroid), centrally within the myometrium (intramural fibroid), at the outer border of the myometrium (subserosal fibroid) or attached to the uterus by a narrow pedicle containing blood vessels (pedunculated fibroid). Cervical fibroids arise from the cervix (Figures 10.1 and 10.2). Fibroids can arise separately from the uterus, especially in the broad ligament, presumably from embryonal remnants. The typical whorled appearance may be altered following degeneration; three forms of which are recognized: red, hyaline and cystic. Fibroids are oestrogen dependent.

Red degeneration follows an acute disruption of the blood supply to the fibroid during active growth, classically during the mid-second trimester of pregnancy. This may present with the sudden onset of pain with localized tenderness to an area of the uterus, associated with a mild pyrexia and leuckocytosis. The symptoms and signs typically resolve over a few days and surgical intervention is rarely required.

Hyaline degeneration occurs when the fibroid gradually outgrows its blood supply, and may

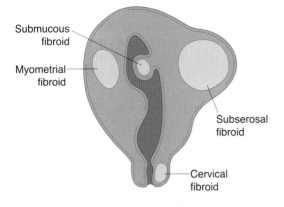

Figure 10.1   Diagram showing typical location of uterine fibroids.

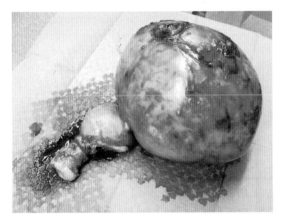

Figure 10.2   Pedunculated fibroid at hysterectomy specimen.

progress to central necrosis, leaving cystic spaces at the centre, termed 'cystic degeneration'. As the final stage in the natural history, calcification of a fibroid may be detected incidentally on an abdominal x-ray in a post-menopausal woman. Rarely, malignant or sarcomatous degeneration can occur but the incidence of this is in 1:200 cases or less. The suspicion is greatest in the post-menopausal period when there is a rapidly increasing size of fibroid.

Clinical features

Fibroids are common. They are present in about 20 per cent of women over 30 years of age. Autopsy studies show a prevalence of up to 50 per cent. Risk factors for clinically significant fibroids are nulliparity,

obesity, a positive family history and African racial origin (three times higher risk). The vast majority of fibroids are asymptomatic, but may be identified coincidentally. Abdominal examination might indicate the presence of a firm mass arising from the pelvis. Unless fibroids cause symptoms they do not require any treatment. Common presenting symptoms are menstrual disturbance and pressure symptoms, especially urinary frequency. Pain is unusual, except in the special circumstance of acute degeneration as discussed above. Menorrhagia usually indicates that the fibroid is of submucous origin which is distorting the endometrial cavity by increasing the endometrial surface area. It has been shown that removal of the submucous component, in the presence of other types of fibroids, resolves the menorrhagia symptoms.

Subfertility may result from mechanical distortion or occlusion of the Fallopian tubes, and an endometrial cavity grossly distorted by submucous fibroids may prevent implantation of a fertilized ovum. Therefore, fibroids do not require removal unless there is proven infertility. Once a pregnancy is established, however, the risk of miscarriage is not increased. In late pregnancy, fibroids located in the cervix or lower uterine segment may cause an abnormal lie. After delivery, postpartum haemorrhage may occur due to inefficient uterine contraction.

Investigations

Often the clinical features alone will be sufficient to establish the diagnosis. A haemoglobin concentration will help to indicate anaemia if there is clinically significant menorrhagia. Ultrasonography is the mainstay of diagnosis to distinguish between a fibroid and an ovarian mass. In the presence of large fibroids, ultrasonography is helpful to exclude hydronephrosis from pressure on the ureters.

Treatment

Conservative management is appropriate where asymptomatic fibroids are detected incidentally. It may be useful to establish the growth rate of the fibroids by repeat clinical examination or ultrasound after a 6–12-month interval. The main types of medical treatment for heavy menstrual bleeding (tranexemic acid, mefenamic acid, combined oral contraceptive pill) tend to be ineffective. The only effective medical treatment is to use gonadotrophin-releasing hormone (GnRH) agonists. Unfortunately, while very effective in shrinking fibroids, when ovarian function returns, the fibroids regrow to their previous dimensions. Therefore, these treatments are usually limited to use in preparation for surgery. Mifepristone (an antiprogestogen) has been shown to be effective in shrinking fibroids at a low dose, but is currently not available for use as it causes endometrial hyperplasia. The optimal dose, duration of treatment and long-term effects have yet to be established.

The choice of surgical treatment is determined by the presenting complaint and the patient's aspirations for menstrual function and fertility. Menorrhagia associated with a submuccous fibroid or fibroid polyp should be treated by hysteroscopic removal (Figure 10.3). Where a bulky fibroid uterus causes pressure symptoms, the options are myomectomy with uterine conservation, or hysterectomy. Myomectomy will be the preferred option where preservation of fertility is required. An important point for the preoperative discussion during the consent process is that there is a small but significant risk of uncontrolled life-threatening bleeding during myomectomy, which could lead to hysterectomy.

Uterine artery embolization (UAE) is a newer technique performed by interventional radiologists. It involves embolization of both uterine arteries under radiological guidance with a small incision in the femoral artery performed under local anaesthesia. The current evidence indicates that the overall shrinkage of fibroids and reduction in menstrual blood loss is around 50 per cent, although long-term follow-up data beyond 18–24 months are not available. Following UAE, patients usually require admission overnight because of pain following arterial occlusion requiring opiate analgesia. Complications include fever, infection, fibroid expulsion and potential ovarian failure. Women wishing to retain their fertility should be counselled carefully before undergoing UAE as the effects are not known, although there have been pregnancies reported in the literature.

Hysterectomy and myomectomy can be facilitated by GnRH agonist pretreatment over a three-month period to reduce the bulk and vascularity of the fibroids. Useful benefits of this approach are to enable a suprapubic (low transverse) rather than a midline abdominal incision, or to facilitate vaginal rather than abdominal hysterectomy, both of which are conducive to more rapid recovery and fewer postoperative complications. GnRH agonist pretreatment can obscure tissue planes around the fibroid making surgery more difficult but, on the positive side, blood loss and the likely need for transfusion are reduced.

Key Points

- Cervical ectropion is a common finding and is usually due to hormonal influence, e.g. three Ps: puberty, pill and pregnancy.

- Fibroids are common, being detectable clinically in about 20 per cent of women over 30 years of age.

- Fibroids are oestrogen dependent and therefore undergo shrinkage after the menopause.

- The vast majority of fibroids are asymptomatic. Only those presenting with symptoms should be treated, i.e. submucous types causing abnormal uterine bleeding.

- Hysteroscopic techniques for the removal of submucous fibroids are successful and avoid major surgery.

- The mechanism whereby fibroids affect fertility is unclear.

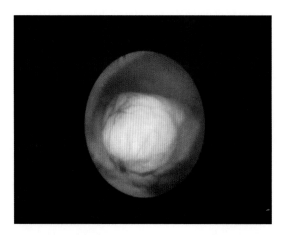

Figure 10.3 Hysteroscopic appearance of a fibroid polyp within the endometrial cavity.

Additional reading

Gupta JK, Sinha A, Lumsden MA, Hickey M. Uterine artery embolization for symptomatic uterine fibroids. *Cochrane Database Syst Rev* 2006; (**1**): CD005073.

Lethaby A, Vollenhoven B, Sowter MC. Pre-operative GnRH analogue therapy before hysterectomy or myomectomy for uterine fibroids. *Cochrane Database Syst Rev* 2001; (**2**): CD000547.

CASE HISTORY

Mrs DBP is a 42-year-old Afro-Caribbean woman who has a large abdominal mass, but no symptoms of heavy periods. The smear history is normal. She has two children but still wishes to retain her fertility as she is planning a third. She is married, a non-smoker and otherwise fit and well. On examination, the abdomen is distended and there is a pelvic mass consistent with that of a 20-week size pregnancy. Vaginal examination confirms this and ultrasound scan shows two large fibroids that are intramyometrial but also subserous.

Discussion

How would you manage this patient?

The important factor here is that Mrs DBP is asymptomatic and therefore there is no need for any specific treatment. The other important feature is that she wishes to retain her fertility and therefore hysterectomy is contraindicated.

Myomectomy is not necessary unless she has problems conceiving. She should be counselled that there is a risk of bleeding and that hysterectomy is a possibility. Uterine artery embolization is another possibility but its effect on future fertility is not completely known. Hysterectomy will give an outstandingly good result as it removes the uterine bulk mass and all future risk of bleeding, but is associated with surgical complications.

ENDOMETRIOSIS AND ADENOMYOSIS

OVERVIEW

Endometriosis remains a challenging condition for clinicians and patients. Difficulties exist in relation to explanation of its aetiology, pathophysiology and progression and to its recognition, both from symptoms and at endoscopy. Similar problems exist in determining who and when to treat and for how long once the diagnosis has been made.

Introduction

Endometriosis is a common condition which is defined as endometrial tissue lying outside the endometrial cavity. It is usually found within the peritoneal cavity, predominantly within the pelvis, commonly on the uterosacral ligaments. It can also be found in other sites such as umbilicus, abdominal scars, nasal passages and pleural cavity.

Endometriotic tissue responds to cyclical hormonal changes and therefore undergoes cyclical bleeding and local inflammatory reaction. Repeated bleeding and healing leads to fibrosis. This cyclical damage causes adhesions between associated organs causing pain and infertility.

Adenomyosis is when there is endometrial tissue found deep within the myometrium. The uterus becomes enlarged and 'boggy' to feel. It causes heavy painful menstruation. Adenomyosis is usually diagnosed post-hysterectomy although magnetic resonance imaging (MRI) can diagnose adenomyosis pre-surgery.

Incidence

Endometriosis occurs in approximately 1–2 per cent of women of reproductive age. It is the most common benign gynaecological condition, estimated to be present in between 10 and 15 per cent of women. It is

a condition that is oestrogen dependent and therefore it resolves after the menopause or when treatment is directed towards inducing a pseudomenopause.

Aetiology

The aetiology of endometriosis is unknown, although there have been many theories. There is, however, unlikely to be a single theory that explains the aetiology of endometriosis:

Menstrual regurgitation and implantation

Sampson's implantation theory postulates retrograde menstrual regurgitation of viable endometrial glands and tissue within the menstrual fluid and subsequent implantation on the peritoneal surface. This has been induced in animal/primate models. Endometriosis is also found in women with genital tract abnormalities where there is obstruction to menstrual fluid.

Coelomic epithelium transformation

Meyer's 'coelomic metaplasia' theory describes the de-differentiation of peritoneal cells lining the Müllerian duct back to their primitive origin which then transform into endometrial cells. This transformation into endometrial cells may be due to hormonal stimuli or inflammatory irritation.

Genetic and immunological factors

It has been suggested that genetic and immunological factors may alter the susceptibility of a woman and allow her to develop endometriosis. There appears to be an increased incidence in first-degree relatives of patients with the disorder and racial differences, with increased incidence among oriental women and a low prevalence in women of Afro-Caribbean origin.

Vascular and lymphatic spread

Vascular and lymphatic embolization to distant sites has been demonstrated and explains the rare findings of endometriosis in sites outside the peritoneal cavity.

Clinical features

Classical clinical features are severe cyclical non-colicky pelvic pain restricted to around the time of menstruation, sometimes associated with heavy menstrual loss. Symptoms may begin a few days before menses starts until the end of menses. It is well recognized that there is a lack of correlation between extent of disease and the intensity of symptoms.

Pelvic pain presenting with colicky pain throughout the menstrual cycle may be associated with irritable bowel syndrome symptoms. Deep pain with intercourse (deep dyspareunia) can also indicate the presence of endometriosis in the pouch of Douglas.

Endometriosis in distant sites can cause local symptoms, for example cyclical epistaxis with nasal passage deposits, cyclical rectal bleeding with bowel deposits (see Table 11.1).

Physical examination

Endometriosis can be suspected by clinical findings on vaginal examination of thickening or nodularity of the uterosacral ligaments, tenderness in the pouch of Douglas, an adnexal mass or a fixed retroverted uterus. However, pelvic tenderness alone is nonspecific, and differential diagnoses for restricted mobility of the uterus include chronic pelvic inflammatory disease and uterine, ovarian or cervical malignancy. In these conditions, other suggestive features are usually present.

Investigations

Ultrasound

Transvaginal ultrasound can detect gross endometriosis involving the ovaries (endometriomas

Table 11.1   Symptoms of endometriosis in relationship to site of lesion

Site	Symptoms
Female reproductive tract	Dsymenorrhoea
	Lower abdominal and pelvic pain
	Dyspareunia
	Rupture/torsion endometrioma
	Low back pain
	Infertility
Urinary tract	Cyclical haematuria/dysuria
	Ureteric obstruction
Gastrointestinal tract	Dyschezia (pain on defecation)
	Cyclical rectal bleeding
	Obstruction
Surgical scars/umbilicus	Cyclical pain and bleeding
Lung	Cyclical haemoptysis
	Haemopneumothorax

or chocolate cysts). In smaller lesions, ultrasound is of limited value. However, the use of ultrasound can be reassuring by excluding gross disease.

Magnetic resonance imaging

MRI can detect lesions >5 mm in size, particularly in deep tissues, for example rectovaginal septum. This can allow careful presurgical planning in difficult cases.

Laparoscopy

Although laparoscopy remains the traditional method for diagnosis, it is based on the accuracy of the visual diagnosis of endometriotic lesions, which is dependent upon the experience of the laparoscopist. The endometriosis lesions can be red, puckered, black 'matchstick' or white fibrous lesions (see Figure 11.1). The advantage of laparoscopy is that it affords concurrent surgical diathermy and/or excision of the endometriotic lesions and also a staging of the disease.

Endometriosis and infertility

It is estimated that between 30 and 40 per cent of patients with endometriosis complain of difficulty in conceiving. In many patients, there is a multifactorial pathogenesis to this subfertility. It has yet to be shown how the presence of a few small endometriotic deposits might render a patient subfertile. In the more severe stages of endometriosis, there is commonly anatomical distortion, with peri-adnexal adhesions and destruction of ovarian tissue when endometriomas develop. A number of possible and variable mechanisms have been postulated to connect mild endometriosis with infertility (Table 11.2).

From the balance of available evidence, medical treatment of endometriosis does not improve fertility and should not be given to patients wishing to conceive. However, surgical ablation/excision of minimal and mild endometriosis does improve fertility chances. Surgical treatment of endometriomas probably increases spontaneous pregnancy rates, including *in vitro* fertilization success rates.

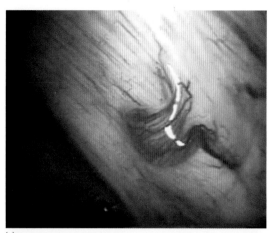

(a)

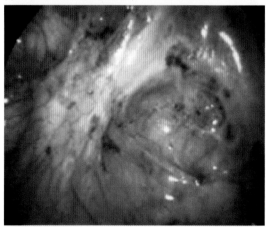

(b)

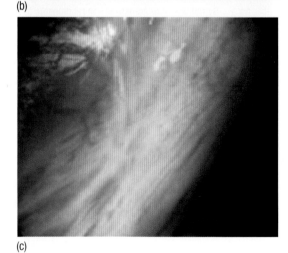

(c)

Figure 11.1 (a) Red lesion on peritoneum; (b) black 'matchstick' lesions; (c) white fibrous lesion.

Table 11.2   Infertility and endometriosis – possible mechanisms

Ovarian function	Luteolysis caused by prostaglandins F2
	Oocyte maturation defects
	Endocrinopathies
	Luteinized unruptured follicle syndrome
	Altered prolactin release
	Anovulation
Tubal function	Impaired fimbrial oocyte pick-up
	Altered tubal mobility
Coital function	Deep dyspareunia – reduced coital frequency
Sperm function	Antibodies causing inactivation
	Macrophage phagocytosis of spematozoa
Early pregnancy failure	Prostaglandin induced
	Immune reaction
	Luteal phase deficiency

Management

Patients with endometriosis are often difficult to treat, not only from a physical point of view, but also often because of associated psychological issues. Therapies designed for long-term strategies should be used. Coexisting additional diseases such as irritable bowel/constipation (present in up to 80 per cent of cases) should also be treated to improve overall success rates. Endometriosis is known to be a recurrent disorder throughout the whole of reproductive life and it is impossible to guarantee complete cure. Treatment should therefore be tailored for the individual according to her age, symptoms, extent of the disease and her desire for future childbearing. In a significant proportion of patients, there is little progression of the disease.

Medical therapy

Analgesics

Non-steroidal anti-inflammatory drugs (NSAIDs) are potent analgesics and are helpful in reducing the severity of dysmenorrhoea and pelvic pain. However, they have no specific impact on the disease and hence their use is for symptom control only. The additional use of codeine/opiates should be avoided as the coexisting irritable bowel symptoms can be worsened, exacerbating pelvic pain symptoms.

Combined oral contraceptive agents

Oral contraceptive agents can be used for diagnostic and therapeutic purposes. After the known risk factors for the suitability of the combined oral contraceptive (COC) are evaluated, COC should be prescribed to be taken continuously for an initial six-month period, to render the patient amenorrhoeic. If symptoms of cyclical pelvic pain disappear (in the absence of any gross endometriosis on ultrasound, e.g. endometrioma), the diagnosis is one of minimal/mild endometriosis. If symptoms persist then there is likely to be coexisting irritable bowel disease/constipation which requires its own treatment strategies of high fibre and adequate fluid intake. If there is symptomatic relief with the continuous use of COC, then this therapy should be continued indefinitely for up to several years or even longer until pregnancy is intended.

Progestogens

In those where there are risk factors for the use of COC, progestogens should be used, for example Cerazette or medroxyprogesterone acetate. As long as amenorrhoea can be induced, symptoms related to endometriosis should be alleviated. The use of levonorgestrel intrauterine systems (LNG-IUS) has been shown to be effective in achieving a long-term therapy effect, particularly after surgical treatment. The effect is probably related to 100 per cent compliance with treatment.

Danazol/gestrinone

The use of danazol and gestrinone, ovarian suppressive agents, are now not commonly used agents. Although effective, side effects, such as androgen effects, for example weight gain, greasy skin and acne over long term (>six months), alterations in lipid profiles or liver function, limit their use.

Gonadotrophin-releasing hormone agonists

Gonadotrophin-releasing hormone agonists (GnRH-A) are as effective as danazol in relieving the severity and symptoms of endometriosis and differ only in their side effects. These drugs induce a state of hypogonadotrophic hypogonadism or pseudo-menopause with low circulating levels of oestrogen. Side effects include symptoms seen at the menopause, in particular hot flushes and night sweats. Despite these side effects, the drugs are well tolerated and they have become established agents in the treatment of endometriosis. They are available as multiple, daily-administered intranasal sprays or as slow-release depot formulations, each lasting for one month or more. Long-term use (>six months) can lead to drug-induced osteoporosis, limiting its use. The administration of low-dose hormone replacement therapy (HRT), along with the GnRH-A analogues, the so-called 'add-back' therapy, may offer a way of preventing the adverse effects of oestrogen deficiency. The recurrence of symptoms on cessation of therapy is usually rapid, therefore the long-term use of GnRH should be restricted to diagnostic purposes and where it is used to suppress menstruation, in addition to using long-term therapy, such as the LNG-IUS system.

Surgical treatment

Conservative surgery

Laparoscopic surgery with techniques such as diathermy, laser vaporization or excision has become the standard for the surgical management of endometriosis. Endometriotic cysts should not just be drained but the inner cyst lining should be excised or destroyed. Recurrent risks following conservative surgery are as high as 30 per cent and therefore concurrent long-term medical therapy is usually useful.

Definitive surgery

Where there are severe symptoms or progressive disease or in women whose families are complete, definitive surgery for the relief of dysmenorrhoea and pain necessitates hysterectomy and bilateral salpingo-oophorectomy, which is usually curative. The removal of the ovaries is essential in achieving long-term symptom relief. The commencement of combined HRT may be deferred for up to six months following surgery, particularly when active disease was found to be present at the time of laparotomy, to prevent activation of any residual disease.

Adenomyosis

Adenomyosis is a disorder in which endometrial glands are found deep within the myometrium. Adenomyosis is increasingly being viewed as a separate pathological entity affecting a different population of patients with an as yet unknown and different aetiology.

Patients with adenomyosis are usually multiparous and diagnosed in their late thirties or early forties. They present with increasingly severe secondary dysmenorrhoea and increased menstrual blood loss (menorrhagia). Examination of patients may be useful with the findings most often of a bulky and sometimes tender 'boggy' uterus, particularly if examined perimenstrually. Ultrasound examination of the uterus may be helpful for diagnosis when adenomyosis is particularly localized showing haemorrhage-filled, distended endometrial glands. Sometimes this may give an irregular nodular development within the uterus, very similar to that of uterine fibroids. MRI is the more definitive investigation of choice as it provides excellent images of the myometrium, endometrium and areas of adenomyosis (see Figure 11.2).

Given the practical difficulty in making the diagnosis of adenomyosis preoperatively, conservative surgery and medical treatments are so far poorly developed. In general, any treatment that induces amenorrhoea will be helpful as it will relieve pain and excessive bleeding. On ceasing treatment, however, the symptoms rapidly return in the majority of patients, and hysterectomy remains the only definitive treatment.

Additional reading

Jacobson TZ, Duffy JMN, Barlow D *et al.* Laparoscopic surgery for subfertility associated with endometriosis. *Cochrane Database Syst Rev* 2002; (**4**): CD001398.

NHS Clinical Knowledge Summaries on Endometriosis. Available from: www.cks.nhs.uk/endometriosis. August 2010.

Royal College of Obstetricians and Gynaecologists. The investigation and management of endometriosis. Green-top Guideline No. 24. October 2006. www.rcog.org.uk/files/rcog-corp/uploaded-files/GT24InvestigationEndometriosis2006.pdf

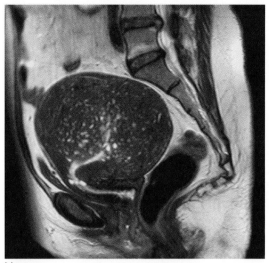

(a)

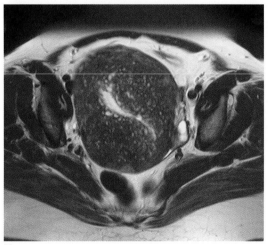

(b)

Figure 11.2   MRI images of adenomyosis.

Key Points

- Endometriosis is one of the most common gynaecological conditions and affects between 10 and 25 per cent of women.

- Endometriosis is oestrogen dependent.

- Endometriosis presents with cyclical non-colicky pelvic pain restricted to around the time of menstruation, sometimes associated with heavy menstrual loss.

- Endometriosis is associated with tubal and ovarian damage and the formation of adhesions and can compromise fertility.

- Medical treatment of endometriosis involves suppressing oestrogen levels to induce amenorrhoea using continuous oral contraceptive pills, progestogens or GnRH agonists.

- The surgical treatment of endometriosis is either minimally invasive, using laparoscopic techniques, or radical, with total abdominal hysterectomy and bilateral salpingo-oophorectomy.

DISEASES OF THE OVARY

OVERVIEW

The ovaries develop from the mesonephric system and maintain a separate vascular system from the rest of the genital tract. Ovarian dysfunction is common and the majority of abnormalities are self-limiting and benign. It is important to note that the risk of ovarian malignancy increases with age. Ovarian cancer is rare in children and adolescents and approximately 5 per cent of ovarian malignancies occur in women less than 20 years old. This chapter will deal with benign and malignant diseases of the ovary.

Benign diseases of the ovary

Benign ovarian tumours are listed in Table 12.1. Most benign ovarian tumours will be diagnosed by the presence of a pelvic/abdominal mass, by symptoms such as pain or incidentally usually on ultrasound. The differential diagnosis of a pelvic mass includes tumours of uterus, Fallopian tube, urinary tract and bowel and pregnancy.

The causes of benign ovarian tumours will vary with age. Functional cysts are common in young girls, adolescents and women in their reproductive years. Germ cell tumours occur more commonly in young women whereas benign epithelial tumours occur more commonly in older women.

Diagnosis may be made by symptoms of pain or pressure on the bowel or bladder. Acute pain may represent torsion of a cyst, rupture or haemorrhage into it. Examination may elicit a pelvic/abdominal mass separate from the uterus.

Common investigations include ultrasound scan (USS) (transvaginal or abdominal), CT scans or magnetic resonance imaging (MRI), as well as tumour markers (see Table 12.2). A pregnancy test should be performed to exclude pregnancy. Inflammatory markers, such as CRP and WCC, are important if the differential diagnosis includes appendicitis or a tubo-ovarian abcess.

Functional ovarian cysts

This group includes follicular, corpus luteal and theca luteal cysts. The risk of developing functional cysts is reduced by the use of the oral contraceptive pill. Little is known about the aetiology, diagnosis is made when the cyst measures more than 3 cm (normal ovulatory follicles measure up to 2.5 cm), they rarely grow larger than 10 cm and appear as simple unilocular cysts on USS. Treatment depends on symptoms, if asymptomatic they can be observed and sequential

Table 12.1 Causes of benign ovarian cysts

Functional	Follicular cyst
	Corpus luteal cyst
	Theca luteal cyst
Inflammatory	Tubo-ovarian abscess
	Endometrioma
Germ cell	Benign teratoma
Epithelial	Serous cystadenoma
	Mucinous cystadenoma
	Brenner tumour
Sex cord stromal	Fibroma
	Thecoma

Table 12.2   Tumour markers used in ovarian carcinoma

Tumour Marker	Tumour type	Uses
Ca 125	Epithelial ovarian cancer (serous), borderline ovarian tumours	Preoperative, follow up
Ca 19-9	Epithelial ovarian cancer (mucinous), borderline ovarian tumours	Preoperative, follow up
Inhibin	Granulosa cell tumours	Follow up
β-hCG	Dysgerminoma, choriocarcinoma	Preoperative, follow up
AFP	Endodermal yolk sack, teratoma	Preoperative, follow up

repeat ultrasound can be performed. If symptomatic, laparoscopic cystectomy may be performed.

Corpus luteal cysts occur following ovulation and may present with pain due to rupture and or haemorrhage, typically late in the menstrual cycle. Treatment is expectant, with analgesia. Occasionally, surgery may be necessary to wash out the pelvis and perform an ovarian cystectomy.

Theca luteal cysts are associated with pregnancy, particularly multiple pregnancy, and are often diagnosed incidentally at routine USS. Most resolve spontaneously during pregnancy.

Inflammatory ovarian cysts

This is usually associated with pelvic inflammatory disease (PID) (see Chapter 6, Genital infections in gynaecology), and is most common in young women. The inflammatory mass may involve the tube, ovary and bowel and can be noted as a mass or an abscess. Occasionally, the tubo-ovarian mass can develop from other infective causes, for example appendicitis or diverticular disease.

Diagnosis is based on that for PID, inflammatory markers are helpful and treatment may include antibiotics, surgical drainage or excision. Definitive surgery is usually deferred until after the acute infection due to increased risk of systemic infection and difficulty with inflamed and infected tissue.

Patients may present with endometriomas, often known as 'chocolate cysts' due to the presence of altered blood within the ovary. They can reach 10 cm in size and have a characteristic 'ground glass' appearance on USS. Further management of endometriosis is discussed in Chapter 11, Endometriosis and adenomyosis.

Germ cell tumours

These are the most common ovarian tumours in young women, peak incidence is in the early 20s accounting for more than 50 per cent of ovarian tumours in this age group. The most common form of benign germ cell tumour is the mature dermoid cyst (cystic teratoma), 80 per cent of these occur during reproductive life. Up to 10 per cent of dermoid cysts can be bilateral. The risk of malignant transformation is rare (<2 per cent), usually occurring in women over 40 years.

Dermoid cysts are a combination of all tissue types (mesenchymal, epithelial and stroma). Diagnosis may be incidental, although 15 per cent present acutely with torsion (Figure 12.1). Torsion cuts off blood supply to the ovarian tissue, presenting symptoms are usually acute onset of pain associated with nausea. Any mature tissue type may be present and often hair, muscle, cartilage, bone or teeth may be noted. Because of the high fat content present in dermoid cysts, MRI is particularly useful in making the diagnosis.

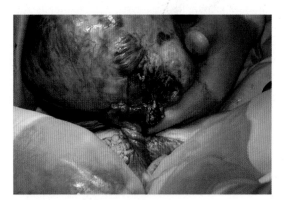

Figure 12.1   Torsion of dermoid cyst.

Treatment is often surgical excision, torsion may require complete oophorectomy. If the ovary is viable then cystectomy can be performed, often laparoscopically.

Epithelial tumours

Benign epithelial tumours increase with age and are most common in peri-menopausal women. The most common epithelial tumours are serous cystadenomas, accounting for 20–30 per cent of benign tumours in women under 40. Typically, serous cystadenomas are unilocular and rarely involve the opposite ovary. Mucinous cystadenomas are large multiloculated cysts and are bilateral in 10 per cent of cases.

Brenner tumours are often small tumours found incidentally within the ovary. They may secrete oestrogen.

Sex cord stromal tumours

Ovarian fibromas are the most common sex cord stromal tumours. They are solid ovarian tumours composed of stromal cells. They present in older women often with torsion due to the heavinesss of the ovary. Occasionally, patients may present with Meig syndrome (pleural effusion, ascites and ovarian fibroma). Following removal of the ovarian fibroma, the pleural effusion will often resolve.

Thecomas are benign oestrogen-secreting tumours. They often present post-menopause with manifestations of excess oestrogen production such as post-menopausal bleeding. Although benign, they may induce an endometrial carcinoma.

Other ovarian cysts

Other cysts occasionally presenting as ovarian tumours include fimbrial cysts, paratubal cysts and other uncommon embryologically derived cysts such as cysts of Morgani.

Malignant ovarian tumours

Introduction

Ovarian cancer is the second most common gynaecological malignancy and the major cause of death from a gynaecological cancer. There are approximately 6000 cases per year within the UK. Unfortunately survival from ovarian cancer remains poor, due in part to the late presentation of the disease. However, if diagnosed in the early stages, survival is equivalent to endometrial cancer. The majority of cancers arise from the ovarian epithelium and occur in older age groups with a mean age of 64 years at presentation.

Surgery and combination chemotherapy are the mainstay of treatment for ovarian cancer. Germ cell tumours are uncommon, usually presenting in a younger age group and are often cured with conservative surgery and chemotherapy with preservation of fertility.

Incidence

The lifetime risk of developing ovarian cancer in the general population is 1.4 per cent (one in 70), mean age of presentation is 64 years. Ovarian cancer is more prevalent in developed nations, there are variations in incidence with ethnicity, Caucasian women have the highest incidence at approximately 14 per 100 000, whereas Asian women have a lower incidence at 10 per 100 000. Ovarian cancer is rare in young women and only 3 per cent of ovarian cancers occur in women under 35 years. It is now becoming increasingly accepted that a large proportion of ovarian cancers originate as Fallopian tube cancers which have spread or implanted into the ovarian epithelium. There is a significant genetic aspect to ovarian cancer (see below). It is recognized that women with hereditary cancer present early, with a mean age at diagnosis of 54 years.

Aetiology and risk factors

Eighty per cent of ovarian cancers are derived from the ovarian epithelium, other cell types include germ cell and sex cord-stromal and are discussed later in the chapter.

Epithelial ovarian cancer is due to malignant transformation of the ovarian epithelium, this is the same as peritoneal mesothelium. The molecular events leading to malignancy remain poorly understood, a number of gene mutations resulting in suppression of tumour suppressor genes, such as p16 and p53, along with overexpression of oncogenes, such as HER2, have been associated with sporadic epithelial ovarian cancer (EOC). There is a recognized association with germline mutations in BRCA1 and BRCA2 genes in hereditary EOC (see below under Genetic factors in ovarian cancer). The process of malignant change is associated with reproduction and ovulation, there are two main theories:

1 Incessant ovulation theory: This relates to continuous ovulation causing repeated trauma to the ovarian epithelium leading to genetic mutation and development of a cancer. This is supported by an increased incidence of EOC in nulliparous women, women with early menarche or late menopause and a reduction in incidence of EOC in multiparous women and in women who have used oral contraception.

2 Excess gonadatrophin secretion: This promotes higher levels of oestrogen which in turn leads to epithelial proliferation and malignant transformation of the ovarian epithelium.

In addition to the risk factors outlined above, further factors influencing the risk of ovarian cancer are found in Table 12.3.

Table 12.3   Risk factors in ovarian cancer

Decreased risk of ovarian cancer	Increased risk of ovarian cancer
Multiparity	Nuliparity
Oral contraceptive pill (RR reduced by 20% per 5 years use)	Intrauterine device (RR 1.76)
Tubal ligation	Endometriosis
Hysterectomy	Cigarette smoking (mucinous tumours only)
	Obesity

Genetic factors in ovarian cancer

It is estimated that at least 10–15 per cent of women with EOC have a genetic link (Pal et al., 2005). There are now at least three known forms of hereditary EOC – BRCA1, BRCA2 and Lynch syndrome. The lifetime risk of ovarian cancer in the general population is one in 70 or 1.4 per cent. This rises to one in 20 or 5 per cent if women have one family member affected and further increases to 40–50 per cent if two first degree relatives are affected. Hereditary cancers usually occur around ten years before sporadic cancers and are associated with other cancers (breast, colorectal).

The most common hereditary cancer in the breast ovarian cancer syndrome (BRCA), accounting for 90

per cent of the hereditary cancers. This syndrome is due to a mutation of tumour suppressor genes, the most common is BRCA1 (80 per cent) and BRCA2 (15 per cent). Lynch syndrome is hereditary non-polyposis colorectal cancer (HNPCC) and is associated with endometrial cancer and a 10 per cent risk of ovarian cancers. Hereditary EOC tend to be adenocarcinomas, present in later stages, and recent evidence supports improved survival, probably due to a better response to platinum chemotherapy (Cass et al., 2003).

Management of women with a family history of ovarian cancer

This depends on the women's age, reproductive plans and individual risk. Ideally, women with a strong family history should be referred to clinical genetics for assessment of the family tree. If the pedigree suggests a hereditary cancer genetic testing for BRCA1 and BRCA2 may be offered. At present, screening is offered to women aged 35 and over. This is usually yearly transvaginal ultrasound and measurement of Ca125, however this strategy is not very sensitive or specific. Prospective studies are being carried out looking at 4–6-monthly measurements of Ca125. Prophylactic bilateral salpingo-oohorectomy has a role in patients who are found to be carrying a gene mutation and have completed their family, although it does not completely eliminate the risk of a primary peritoneal tumour.

Classification of ovarian cancer

Primary ovarian tumours can originate from the epithelium, the connective tissue of the ovary (sex cord stromal) or the germ cells. In addition, the ovary is a common site for metastatic tumours, including Krukenberg tumours, common sites include colon, stomach and breast. Table 12.4 shows a histological classification of ovarian tumours.

Epithelial tumours of the ovary can be benign, malignant or borderline. Approximately 10 per cent of epithelial tumours are classified as borderline tumours. These tumours are well differentiated with some features of malignancy but are characterized by not invading the basement membrane, borderline tumours can spread to other structures (peritoneum, omentum) and rarely recur following initial surgery. The majority of borderline tumours are serous, mucinous borderline tumours may arise from the large bowel (appendix) and can be associated with pseudomxyoma peritonei.

Table 12.4   Classification of malignant ovarian tumours

1	Epithelial ovarian tumours (80%)	Serous Mucinous Endometroid Clear cell Undifferentiated
2	Sex cord stromal tumours (10%)	Granulosa cell Sertoli–Leydig Gynandroblastoma
3	Germ cell tumours (10%)	Dysgerminoma Endodermal sinus (yolk sac) Teratoma Choriocarcinoma Mixed
4	Metastatic (including Krukenberg tumours)	

Table 12.5   FIGO staging system

Stage	FIGO definition
I	Growth limited to ovaries
IA	Limited to one ovary: no external tumour, capsule intact, no ascites
IB	Limited to both ovaries: no external tumour, capsule intact, no ascites
IC	Either IB or IB, but tumour on surface of ovary or with capsule ruptured or with ascites positive for tumour cells
II	Growth limited to pelvis
IIA	Extension and or metastases to uterus or tubes
IIB	Extension to other pelvic organs
IIIC	As IIA or IIB, but tumour on surface of ovary or with capsule ruptured or with ascites positive for tumour cells
III	Growth limited to abdominal peritoneum or positive retroperitoneal or inguinal lymph nodes
IIIA	Tumour grossly limited to pelvis with negative nodes, but histologically confirmed microscopic peritoneal implants
IIIB	Abdominal implants <2 cm in diameter
IIIC	Abdominal implants >2 cm diameter or positive retroperitoneal or inguinal lymph nodes
IV	Growth involving one or both ovaries with distant metastases Must have positive cytology on pleural effusion, liver parenchyma.

Staging of ovarian cancer

Ovarian cancer staging is based on clinico-pathological assessment, and like other gynaecocolocial cancers uses the FIGO staging system (Table 12.5). Overall, 25 per cent of patients present with stage I disease, 10 per cent stage II, 50 per cent stage III and 15 per cent stage IV disease. Metastatic spread is by direct spread to peritoneum and other organs and by lymphatic spread to pelvic and para-aortic nodes. A high percentage of women with advanced disease have evidence of peritoneal disease on the diaphragmatic peritoneum (Figure 12.2). Women with early ovarian cancer (stage 1–2) have up to 20 per cent metastatic spread to lymph nodes and this rises to 60 per cent in advanced disease (stage III–IV).

Epithelial ovarian cancer

Clinical features of epithelial ovarian cancer

Most women diagnosed with EOC have symptoms, however these symptoms are nonspecific and often

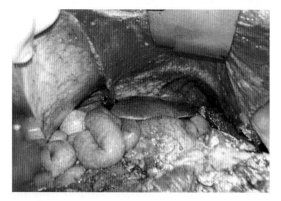

Figure 12.2   Advanced ovarian cancer illustrating diaphragmatic peritoneal disease.

vague. The difficulty with clinical diagnosis is the main reason that patients with ovarian carcinoma present with late stage disease (66 per cent present with stage III disease or greater), this has a dramatic effect on survival. The most common symptoms are:

- persistent pelvic and abdominal pain;
- increased abdominal size/persistent bloating;
- difficulty eating and feeling full quickly.

Other symptoms such as change in bowel habit, urinary symptoms, back ache, irregular bleeding and fatigue occur frequently and any women with persistence of these symptoms should be assessed by their GP.

Strategies, such as population screening, are being assessed in clinical trials to try and improve earlier diagnosis and thus improve survival from ovarian cancer. A large prospective screening study is assessing the role of screening tests in a group of randomly selected post-menopausal women (United Kingdom Collaborative Trial on Ovarian Cancer Screening – UKCTOCS). Early results are promising (Menon *et al.*, 2009) and this important trial will determine if screening can reduce mortality from ovarian cancer and assess the health economics of screening. Until UKCTOCS is completed there is no role for general population screening outside clinical trials.

Examination and investigations

Pelvic and abdominal examination may reveal a fixed, hard mass arising from the pelvis. The differential diagnosis include, non-EOC ovarian cancer, tubo-ovarian abscess, endometriomas or fibroids. In combination with the presence of ascites, a diagnosis of ovarian cancer is highly likely. Early stage ovarian cancer is difficult to diagnose due to the position of the ovary, an adenexal mass may be palpated, it should be noted that less than 20 per cent of adenexal masses palpated in pre-menopausal women are found to be malignant, in post-menopausal women this increases to around 50 per cent.

Chest examination is important to assess pleural fluid and the neck and groin should be examined for enlarged nodes.

Full blood count, urea and electrolytes, liver function tests and chest x-ray are essential. Any suspected pelvic tumour should have measurement of tumour markers, Ca125 is the most common and

is elevated in over 80 per cent of EOC (Table 12.2). USS is the most useful noninvasive test of a suspected malignancy. USS characterizes the morphology of the cyst, presence of bilateral tumours, ascites and omental deposits. In conjunction with Ca125 measurement and age, a risk of malignancy (RMI) score can be calculated.

Approximately 10 per cent of women with EOC will have a synchronous endometrial cancer, it is important to assess the endometrium, especially if conservative surgery is to be undertaken.

If the patient presents with gross ascites or pleural effusion, paracentesis or pleural aspiration may be required. Other investigations that may be needed are CT scan or MRI of abdomen, barium enema or colonoscopy if bowel symptoms are present or there is a possibility of a primary colorectal tumour. If the diagnosis is uncertain or if primary chemotherapy is being considered (for advanced disease, or in patients not fit to undergo surgery), a biopsy may be needed. This can be performed laparoscopically or image guided (USS or CT).

Management of EOC

Surgery

Provided the patient is fit to undergo anaesthetic, surgery remains necessary for diagnosis, staging and treatment of EOC. If the patient is suspected of having ovarian cancer, the surgery should only be performed by a gynaecological oncologist. The objective of surgery is to accurately stage the disease and remove all visible tumour. This is vitally important in ovarian cancer as many studies indicate that the most important prognostic factor is no residual disease following laparotomy.

A vertical incision is required to gain access to all areas of the abdomen. Ascites or peritoneal washings are sampled and a total abdominal hysterectomy and bilateral salping-oophorectomy performed along with an infracolic omentectomy. Further debulking may be required, possibly including resection of bowel, peritoneal stripping or splenectomy in order to remove all tumour. Lymph node resection is important, particularly in early stage disease where studies have found occult metastatic disease in nodes in up to 25 per cent of patients with stage I disease who underwent further surgical staging. Complete debulking to no visible disease varies from 40 to 80 per cent of cases. Often in advanced EOC, there is diffuse spread of disease throughout the abdominal cavity making surgical clearance of tumour very difficult.

If a patient has been operated on outside a cancer centre and is found to have an ovarian cancer, restaging should be offered and this may be carried out laparoscopically. Occasionally, young patients who are found to have an early stage EOC will wish to have conservative, fertility-sparing surgery. In these cases, unilateral salpingo–oophorectomy, omentectomy, peritoneal biopsies and pelvic/paraortic node dissection can be performed with endometrial sampling to exclude a synchronous tumour. Fertility-sparing surgery may also be performed in patients with borderline tumours if fertility is an issue, otherwise pelvic clearance should be performed. If a patient is unfit or unwilling to have surgery, primary chemotherapy may be offered. If the patient responds to the chemotherapy, interval surgery can be carried out after 3–6 cycles. Recent studies indicate that this strategy may reduce postoperative morbidity but does not influence survival. Similarly, if bulky disease remains after surgery and there is a response to chemotherapy, interval debulking may be offered.

Second look surgery is a planned laparotomy at the end of chemotherapy. The main function is to assess and resect any residual disease. Data on second look surgery indicate no survival benefit and consequently it is not standard management outside clinical trials.

Following surgery, all patients with a diagnosis of EOC should be discussed at a gynaecological oncology multidisciplinary team (MDT) meeting where their history, surgical management and histology are reviewed by gynaecological oncologists, oncologists, radiologists, pathologists and nursing staff. If the cancer has been properly staged as stage IA or B, and is histologically low grade (well or moderately differentiated), chemotherapy may be withheld, the role of chemotherapy in stage IC is uncertain, but in practice most patients will be offered postoperative chemotherapy as with all other stages of EOC.

Histology of EOC

Serous adenocarcinomas account for around 75 per cent of all EOC, mucinous and endometroid are less common, accounting for 10 per cent each followed by clear cell and undifferentiated carcinomas. Serous tumours are often poorly differentiated and histologically are characterized by concentric rings of calcification, known as 'psammoma bodies'. Mucinous carcinomas are generally large tumours, with a mean size of 20 cm, multiloculated and can be associated with pseudomxyoma peritonei. Endometroid carcinomas are similar to endometrial cancer, they are associated with endometriosis in approximately 10 per cent of cases and also a synchronous separate endometrial cancer in 10–15 per cent of cases. They tend to be well differentiated and have a better survival compared to serous carcinoma. Clear cell cancer can also arise from endometriosis and are characterized by clear cells similar to renal cancer.

Chemotherapy

Chemotherapy can be given as primary treatment, as an adjunct following surgery or for relapse of disease. It can be used to prolong clinical remission and survival or for palliation. First-line treatment is usually a combination of a platinum compound with paclitaxel. Most regimes are given on an outpatient basis, 3 weeks apart for six cycles.

Platinum compounds are the most effective chemotherapeutic agents in ovarian cancer. They are heavy metal agents that cause cross linkage of DNA strands thus arresting cell replication. Carboplatin is now the main platinum compound used as it is less renal toxic and causes less nausea than cisplatin, but is equally as effective. The dose of carboplatin is calculated according to the glomerular filtration rate (GFR) using the area under the curve (AUC).

Paclitaxol is derived from the bark of the Pacific yew and works by causing microtubular damage to the cell. This prevents replication and cell division. Pre-emptive steroids are given due to high sensitivity reactions, side effects of peripheral neuropathy, neutropenia and myalgia are common and dose dependent. Paclitaxol causes loss of total body hair, irrespective of dose.

Following completion of chemotherapy, patients may have a further CT scan to assess response to treatment. This scan can be used for comparison in the future if there is clinical or biochemical evidence of recurrence.

Follow up of patients includes clinical examination and Ca125 measurement. Studies have shown that levels of Ca125 start to rise prior to onset of clinical evidence of disease, however treating before there is evidence of disease does not improve survival. When disease recurs treatment is largely palliative. If the duration of remission is more than six months, carboplatin may be used, otherwise taxol can be given or other chemotherapy agents, such as topotecan or liposomal doxyrubicin.

Survival from EOC

The survival figures depend on stage at presentation, volume of disease following surgery and the histological grade of tumour. The overall five-year survival from ovarian cancer is 38 per cent in the UK (2001–2006). The figures have improved due to the widespread introduction of centralized MDT care. Survival is stage dependent, overall five-year survival for stage I disease is over 70 per cent compared to 30 per cent for stage III disease. Within stage 1 disease, five-year survival can vary from 95 per cent in a well-differentiated stage IA to 70 per cent for poorly differentiated stage IC tumour. Prognostic factors in ovarian cancer survival are listed in Table 12.6 and Table 12.7 shows the five-year survival rates by stage at diagnosis.

Table 12.6   Prognostic factors in ovarian cancer

Prognostic factors in ovarian cancer
Stage of disease
Volume of residual disease post-surgery
Histological type and grade of tumour
Age at presentation

Table 12.7   Ovarian cancer survival by stage at diagnosis

FIGO stage	5-year survival (%)
I	70–90
II	80
III	30
IV	10–20

Primary peritoneal carcinoma

Primary peritoneal carcinoma (PPC) arises from the peritoneal lining, this tumour type is histologically indistinct from serous ovarian carcinoma. There are, however, morphological differences between the two groups based on clinical findings at laparotomy. Criteria for diagnosis includes:

- normal sized ovaries;

- more extra-ovarian disease than ovarian disease;
- mainly serous histology;
- low volume peritoneal disease.

Using these criteria around 15–20 per cent of EOC are reclassified as PPC, the pattern of spread is similar to EOC and treatment is the same, although there is a trend towards primary chemotherapy as complete surgical debulking is difficult.

Fallopian tube carcinoma

Fallopian tube cancer is a rare cancer, accounting for less than 1 per cent of gynaecological malignancies, however recent studies have hypothesized that the incidence is much higher and a large proportion of EOC are in fact due to metastatic Fallopian tube carcinoma. This is based on the presence of premalignant and malignant changes within the tubes when examined alongside ovarian cancer. The rarity of 'primary Fallopian tube cancer' may be due to tumours that have not metastasized to the ovaries. The clinical diagnosis, investigation and treatment of Fallopian tube cancer is the same as for EOC.

Sex cord stromal tumours

These tumours account for approximately 10 per cent of ovarian tumours, but account for 90 per cent of all functional (i.e. hormone producing) tumours. Generally, they are tumours of low malignant potential with a good long-term prognosis. Some morbidity may arise from the increased oestrogen production (granulose, theca or Sertoli cell) or androgen (Seroli-Leydig or steroid cell) causing precocious puberty, abnormal menstrual bleeding and an increased risk of uterine cancer. The peak incidence is around the menopause, the exception is juvenile granulosa cell tumour, commonly presenting in girls under ten years of age and causing precocious puberty. Overall, granulosa cell tumours are the most common sex cord stromal cell tumours accounting for over 70 per cent of sex cord stromal tumours.

Presentation

A significant percentage of these tumours present with manifestations of their hormone production, commonly as irregular menstrual bleeding, post-menopausal bleeding or precocious puberty in young girls. Granulosa cell tumours may present as a large pelvic mass or with pain due to torsion/haemorrhage.

Sertoli–Leydig cell tumours produce androgens in over 50 per cent of cases. Patients present with a pelvic mass and signs of virilization. Common symptoms are amenorrhoea, deep voice and hirsuitism. Occasionally, this group of tumours can also produce oestrogen and rarely rennin-causing hypertension.

Most sex cord tumours present as unilateral ovarian masses, measuring up to 15 cm in diameter. Histologically, the tumour is often solid with areas of haemorrhage, the cut surface may be yellow due to high levels of steroid production.

Granulosa cell tumours produce inhibin, which can be used for follow-up surveillance, levels often rise prior to clinical detection of recurrence.

Treatment

This is based on the patient's age and wish to preserve fertility. If young, unilateral salpingo-oophorectomy, uterine sampling and staging is sufficient. In the older group, full surgical staging is recommended. Granulosa cell tumours can recur many years after initial presentation and long-term follow up is required. Recurrence is usually well defined and surgery is the mainstay of treatment as there is no effective chemotherapy regime.

Germ cell tumours

Malignant germ cell tumours occur mainly in young women and account for approximately 10 per cent of ovarian tumours. They are derived from primordial germ cells within the ovary and because of this may contain any cell type. The emphasis of management is based mainly on fertility preserving surgery and chemotherapy, often with preservation of fertility.

The most common presenting symptoms are a pelvic mass, 10 per cent present acutely with torsion or haemorrhage and due to the age incidence some present during pregnancy. Seventy per cent of germ cell tumours are stage I; spread is by lymphatics or blood-borne.

Dysgerminomas account for 50 per cent of all germ cell tumours, they are bilateral in 20 per cent of cases and will occasionally secrete βhCG. Endodermal sinus yolk sac tumours are the second most common germ cell tumours accounting for 15 per cent of all germ cell tumours, they are rarely bilateral and will secrete α-fetoprotein (AFP). They present with a large solid mass which will often present acutely with torsion or rupture, spread of endodermal sinus tumours is a late event and is often to the lungs. Immature teratomas account for 15–20 per cent of malignant germ cell tumours and about 1 per cent of all teratomas. They are classified as mature or immature depending on the grading of neural tissue present. About one-third of teratomas will secrete AFP. Occasionally, there can be malignant transformation of a cell type within a mature teratoma. The most common cell type to transform is the epithelium, usually squamous cell carcinoma.

Non-gestational choriocarcinomas are very rare, usually presenting in young girls with irregular bleeding and very high levels of βhCG.

Presentation

Germ cell tumours should be suspected if a young woman presents with a large solid ovarian mass which may be rapidly growing. Tumour markers as detailed in Table 12.2 should be taken preoperatively as this may influence the need for postoperative chemotherapy. MRI is helpful to assess morphology, particularly within teratomas, CT scan of the abdomen allows assessment of the liver and lymph nodes. All patients should have a chest x-ray to exclude pulmonary metastases.

Management of malignant germ cell tumours

Surgery is tailored to suit the patient. As most women presenting with a malignant germ cell tumour will still be within reproductive years, there may be a need to preserve fertility. An exploratory laparotomy is performed to remove the tumour, assess contralateral spread to the other ovary (20 per cent in dysgerminoma). If there is a cyst present, this should be removed. Careful inspection of the abdominal cavity is required with peritoneal biopsies and sampling of any enlarged pelvic or para-aortic nodes performed. If metastatic disease is found, it should be debulked at surgery, frozen sections may be required to assess nodal status.

Postoperative chemotherapy depends on stage of disease. Stage I dysgerminomas and low-grade teratomas are treated by surgery alone and the five-year survival is in excess of 90 per cent. For the remainder of tumours and for patients with disease outside the ovary, chemotherapy is given. The most common regime used is a combination of cisplatin, bleomycin and etoposide (BEP), given as a course of three to four treatments 3 weeks apart. This regime gives long-term cure rates of over 90 per cent and also preserves fertility if required.

If the patient has recurrent disease, 90 per cent will usually present in the first year following diagnosis, salvage chemotherapy has very good success.

References

Cass I, Baldwin RL, Varkey T *et al.* Improved survival in women with BRCA associated ovarian carcinoma. *Cancer* 2003; **97**: 2187–95.

Pal T, Permuth-Wey J, Betts JA *et al.* BRCA1 and BRCA2 mutations account for a large proportion of ovarian carcinoma cases. *Cancer* 2005; **104**: 2807–16.

Menon U, Gentry-Maharaj A, Hallett R *et al.* Sensitivity and specificity of multimodal and ultrasound screening for ovarian cancer, and stage distribution of detected cancer. The results of the prevalence screen of the UK Collaborative Trial of Ovarian Cancer Screening (UKCTOCS) *Lancet Oncol* 2009; **10**: 327–40.

Additional Reading

Barakat RR, Bevers MW, Gershenson DM, Hoskins WJ (eds). *Handbook of gynecologic oncology*, 2nd edn. London: Dunitz, 2002.

Chitrathara K, Rajaram S, Maheswari A (eds). *Ovarian cancer, contemporary and current management.* Delhi: Jaypee, 2009.

Key Points

- Benign ovarian tumours are common throughout reproductive life, risk of malignancy increases with age. Treatment is based on symptoms and size of tumour.

- Epithelial ovarian carcinomas account for 80 per cent of ovarian malignancies, mean age of presentation is 64 years, 10–15 per cent of these cancers are hereditary, presenting at a younger age.

- Symptoms of EOC are ill defined and as a result most present with advanced disease.

- Treatment is based on removing all tumour surgically and combination chemotherapy.

- Survival from EOC is stage dependent, stage I disease has a 70–90 per cent five-year survival, whereas stage III disease has 30 per cent five-year survival.

- Sex cord stromal tumours often present with endocrine effects due to excess secretion of oestrogen and or androgens

- Germ cell tumours present in young women, they are often cured by fertility-preserving surgery and or chemotherapy.

CHAPTER 13

MALIGNANT DISEASE OF THE UTERUS

OVERVIEW

Endometrial cancer is now the most common gynaecological malignancy worldwide and the fourth most common female cancer after breast, colon and lung. The incidence of uterine cancer is increasing because of increasing age of the population, use of hormone replacement therapy (HRT) and obesity. Most endometrial cancer presents in early stages due to abnormal bleeding and the mainstay of management remains surgical. The overall five-year survival rate is around 80 per cent.

Introduction

The most common type of cancer affecting the uterus is adenocarcinoma, this arises from the lining (endometrium) of the uterus, there are two distinct types: endometrioid adenocarcinoma (type 1)and serous papillary carcinoma (type 2). These cancers are very different: type 1 cancers account for 90 per cent of endometrial adenocarcinomas, are oestrogen dependent, occur in younger women and have a good prognosis, whilst type 2 cancers occur in elderly women, are non-oestrogen dependent and have a much poorer prognosis (Figure 13.1). Clear cell carcinoma can rarely arise from the endometrium. In addition to endometrial adenocarcinomas, malignancy can arise from the stroma or myometrium (sarcoma).

Incidence

Endometrial cancers account for approximately 30 per cent of all gynaecological malignancies, the age-related incidence is 95 per 100 000 women. The

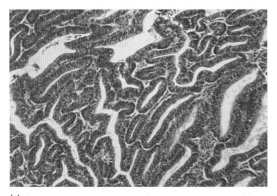
(a)

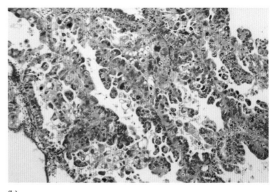
(b)

Figure 13.1 Histological comparison of endometrial adenocarcinom (a) with endometrial serous carcinoma (b).

life-time risk of developing endometrial cancer is approximately one in 90. The mean age of diagnosis is 54, although cancers can be diagnosed in women throughout their reproductive life. The incidence of endometrial cancer rises sharply in the mid 40s, it should be remembered that 25 per cent of cancers occur before the menopause.

Aetiology

The exact causes of endometrial cancer remain unclear, however there is a clear association with high circulating levels of oestrogen; many of the known risk factors (see Table 13.1) relate to high oestrogen levels. In post-menopausal women, conversion of androgens to oestrogen occurs in adipose tissue, there is also interaction with insulin-like growth factor and insulin and endometrial cancer is more common in diabetic patients. Tamoxifen, a selective oestrogen receptor modulator (SERM) used to prevent recurrent breast cancer by blocking oestrogen receptors in the breast, is known to increase the risk of endometrial cancer by up to a factor of 2.5. This is most likely due to a weak oestrogenic effect on the endometrium. New generation SERMs, such as raloxifene, have a lesser or no effect on the endometrium. Genetic causes of endometrial cancer are becoming increasingly more important as genetic services and tests develop. The most common genetic link is with hereditary non-polyposis colorectal cancer syndrome (HNPCC), an autosomal dominant inheritance resulting in mutation of mismatch repair genes MLH1, MSH2 and MSH6. HNPCC is associated with colorectal, ovarian, endometrial and urothelial tumours, the cumulative cancer risk for endometrial cancer varies from 25 to 70 per cent depending on the mutation.

Table 13.1   Risk factors for endometrial cancer

Obesity
Diabetes
Nulliparous
Late menopause >52 years
Unopposed oestrogen therapy
Tamoxifen therapy
Hormone replacement therapy
Family history of colorectal or ovarian cancer

Use of the oral contraceptive pill or progesterone only pill reduces the incidence of endometrial cancer by up to 50 per cent, this appears to be long lasting, smoking also reduces the risk, probably due to the anti-oestrogenic effects of tobacco.

Clinical features

The most common symptom of endometrial cancer is abnormal vaginal bleeding, 90 per cent of patients present with either post-menopausal bleeding (PMB) or irregular vaginal bleeding. Any case of post-menopausal bleeding must be investigated. Audits reveal that upwards of 10 per cent of women with PMB will have a gynaecological malignancy. Common symptoms in pre-menopausal women include intermenstrual bleeding (IMB), blood-stained vaginal discharge, heavy menstrual bleeding (HMB), lower abdominal pain or dyspareunia.

Very rarely, endometrial cancer can be diagnosed by the presence of abnormal glandular cytology at the time of a cervical smear. This often triggers further investigations which diagnose the cancer.

In advanced cancer, patients may present with evidence of fistula, bony metastases, altered liver function or respiratory symptoms.

Diagnosis

At examination, blood may be noted arising from the cervix on speculum examination. Bimanual examination of the uterus may reveal an enlarged uterus. Due to the high risk of endometrial cancer in women with PMB, dedicated clinics may be set up to see and investigate patients urgently. The mainstays of diagnosis are ultrasound scanning, endometrial biopsy and hysteroscopy.

Transvaginal ultrasound scans (TVS) are often performed in the outpatient clinic and allow a quick and accurate assessment of endometrial thickness and of the ovaries (Figure 13.2). Generally, if the endometrium measures less than 4 mm, cancer is very unlikely, any measurement more than this will require hysteroscopy and biopsy. Hysteroscopy can be performed in the outpatient setting or as an inpatient under general anaesthetic. Hysteroscopy allows direct visualization of the whole endometrium and allows a directed biopsy to be performed (Figure

13.3). Endometrial cancer can only be diagnosed by histological examination of a biopsy, endometrial biopsy can be performed using an endometrial sampler, such as the Pipelle, or by curettage. The histological report should give information on cancer type and grade of tumour (i.e. grade 1–3, with 3 equating to high grade). This information is essential as all patients diagnosed with endometrial cancer should be discussed within a gynaecological multidisciplinary meeting to decide on optimal surgical and/or oncology management.

Following a diagnosis of endometrial cancer, magnetic resonance imaging (MRI) is often performed. This will give useful information regarding the extent of disease (stage) and helps to decide on the type of surgical treatment offered to the patient (Figure 13.4).

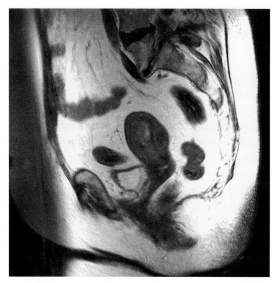

Figure 13.4   MRI of stage 1b endometrial carcinoma.

Staging

The FIGO classification of staging is given in Table 13.2. although this is a surgical classification, patients with low-grade endometrial tumours who are staged as 1a or 1B on MRI may be offered surgery in a cancer unit, whereas all high-grade tumours or those staged >1B should have surgery in a cancer centre.

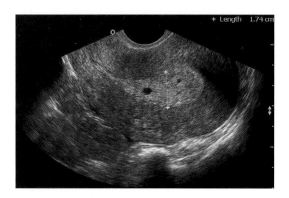

Figure 13.2   Transvaginal ultrasound of the uterus showing thickened endometrium.

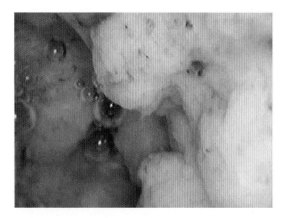

Figure 13.3   Hysteroscopic picture of endometrial carcinoma.

Table 13.2   FIGO staging of carcinoma of the uterus (2009)

1	**Confined to uterine body**
1a	Less than 50% invasion
1b	More than 50% invasion
2	**Tumour invading cervical stroma**
3	**Local and or regional spread of tumour**
3a	Invades serosa of uterus
3b	Invades vagina and/or parametrium
3c	Metastases to pelvic and/or para aortic nodes
4	**Tumour invades bladder ± bowel ± distant metastases**

Management

Surgery

As the majority of patients present with stage 1 disease, surgery is the most common treatment for endometrial cancer. The extent of surgery will depend on a number of factors including; grade of disease, MRI stage and the patient's comorbidities.

The standard surgery is a total hysterectomy, bilateral sapingectomy. This can be performed abdominally or laparoscopically (total, vaginally assisted or robotically). If the patient is low grade (grades 1–2) or MRI staging suggests disease less than stage 1B, then this surgery is adequate. If MRI staging suggests cervical involvement, a radical hysterectomy with pelvic node dissection can be performed (Figure 13.5). If the tumour is high grade (grade 3) or papillary serous, many centres will perform pelvic and para-aortic node dissection as the risk of nodal disease (to either pelvis or para-aortic chain) can be as high

as 30 per cent. The role of nodal dissection remains contentious, a large scale UK study (ASTEC) failed to show a survival benefit in endometrial cancer patients who had pelvic node dissection. Critics of the study highlight that almost 50 per cent of nodal metastases spread to the para-aortic chain and several studies have illustrated survival benefits for patients having pelvic and para-aortic dissection performed.

Adjuvant treatment

Postoperative radiotherapy will reduce the local recurrence rate but does not influence survival. Different units may treat following surgery or wait and treat if the cancer recurs. Strategies for treatment include local radiotherapy to the vaginal vault given over a short period of time (high-dose radiotherapy, HDR), external beam radiotherapy given for locally advanced disease (stage 3) in combination with HDR. Chemotherapy may also be given for metastatic disease to combat the risk of distant spread of the cancer.

Prognosis

The overall five-year survival rate for endometrial cancer is 80 per cent, there is considerable variation in this depending on tumour type, stage and grade of tumour. In stage 1 disease, overall five-year survival ranges from 66 per cent in patients with high-grade 1B disease to 93 per cent for patients with low-grade 1A disease. Overall survival figures are given in Table 13.3.

Table 13.3   Five-year survival for women with endometrial cancer

Stage	5-year survival (%)
I	88
II	75
III	55
IV	16

Adverse prognostic features for survival include advanced age >70 years, high BMI, grade 3 tumours, papillary serous or clear cell histology, lympho-vascular space involvement, nodal metastases and distant metastases.

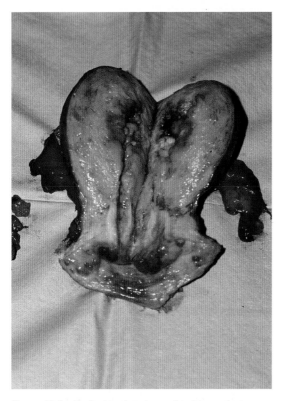

Figure 13.5   Radical hysterectomy showing cervical invasion of endometrial cancer.

Sarcomas of the uterus

These are rare tumours accounting for approximately 5 per cent of all uterine cancers. They are classified into pure sarcomas, heterologous sarcomas or mixed epithelial sarcomas depending on tissue type present in the histological specimen. The most common types are carcinosarcoma or leiomyosarcoma

Pure sarcomas

This group includes endometrial stromal sarcomas (ESS) and leiomyosarcoma. ESS typically occur in perimenopausal women between 45 and 50 years, presenting with irregular bleeding and a soft, enlarged uterus. The majority are low grade and surgery is the main treatment. Leiomyosarcomas are rare tumours of the uterine smooth muscle (myometrium). Rarely (0.75 per cent), they are associated with benign fibroids, usually presenting with a rapidly growing pelvic mass and pain. Preoperative diagnosis is difficult, but may be aided by MRI which can delineate areas of necrosis within the fibroid. The uterus is often enlarged and soft on palpation. Surgery is the main treatment and adjuvant treatment may be considered if the mitotic count is high (above ten mitoses per high powered field). Metastatic spread is usually vascular to distant sites, such as lung and brain.

Mixed epithelial sarcomas (carcinosarcoma)

This group of tumours, formerly known as mixed mesenchymal tumours contain both carcinoma and sarcoma. The carcinomatous element is usually glandular and the sarcomatous element may be endometrial, stromal or occasionally bone, cartilage or muscle. The majority present post-menopausally and occasionally there is a previous history of pelvic radiation. There is usually a history of PMB and a fleshy mass is often seen protruding from the cervix along with an enlarged soft uterus. Treatment is surgery followed by postoperative radiotherapy, five-year survival is 73 per cent if confined to the uterus, but only 25 per cent if the tumour has spread outside the uterus.

Heterologous sarcomas

This rare group of tumours consists of sarcomatous tissue not usually found in the uterus, such as striated muscle, bone or cartilage. The most common is rhabdomyosarcoma which may present in children as a grape-like mass protruding from the cervix with a watery discharge. Histology reveals primitive rhabdomyoblasts. Recurrence rates are high with distant metastases.

Key Points

- Carcinoma of the uterus is the most common gynaecological malignancy.

- The majority of cancers present with stage 1 disease, overall five-year survival is 80 per cent.

- Hyperoestrogen states and obesity play a major aetiological role.

- The majority of patients present with post-menopausal bleeding; however, 25 per cent of cases occur in pre-menopausal women. Endometrial biopsy ± hysteroscopy is the gold standard for diagnosis, whilst MRI may aid in deciding the extent and radicality of surgery.

- Total hysterectomy and bilateral salpingo-oophorectomy is the treatment of choice, pelvic and para-aortic node dissection may be added in advanced disease or in patients with high-grade cancer on endometrial biopsy.

CHAPTER 14

PREMALIGNANT AND MALIGNANT DISEASE OF THE CERVIX

OVERVIEW

The main burden of cervical cancer is in the developing world, where it is a common killer of women in the reproductive age group. This 'hidden' cancer can take away young mothers who are often at the head of the family unit causing considerable emotional and economic upset. In the developed world, the picture is vastly different where cervical cancer is an uncommon cancer thanks to screening, education and access to good medical care. This chapter covers both the pre-invasive and invasive aspects of the disease.

Premalignant disease of the cervix

Introduction

Cervical cancer screening is effective and has contributed to the fall in the developed world of cervical cancer deaths. In the UK, screening has prevented up to 70 per cent of cervical cancer deaths since its inception in 1988.

Human papillomavirus (HPV) infection leads to premalignant change in the cervical epithelium (cervical intraepithelial neoplasia, CIN) which has the potential to turn malignant without treatment. Although not a perfect test, screening the general population with cervical smears has the potential to pick up high-grade disease and this intervention prevents cancer developing.

Epidemiology and aetiology

Infection with the human papilloma virus (HPV) and smoking have been implicated in the development of premalignant and malignant change in the cervix. HPV infection is a sexually transmitted infection spread by skin-to-skin contact during intercourse (condoms do not protect from infections). HPVs are a large family of over 100 different virus types with some (e.g. types 6, 11, 16, 18, 31, 33) having a preference for genital skin. Whereas types 6 and 11 cause genital warts, types 16, 18, 31 and 33 have oncogenic, i.e. cancer-causing properties. Infection is very common with the onset

of sexual activity with up to 80 per cent of sexually active adults showing serological evidence of previous infection. Fortunately, infection is usually transient and of no clinical consequence, but a minority of patients retain the oncogenic viruses within their genital epithelium which can lead to the development of CIN and possible cancer (see below under Natural history of CIN). The role of smoking is unclear, but is likely to be related to the immunosuppressive effects of nicotine derivatives within the cervix which may act as a cofactor with HPV in triggering the development of CIN. Immunosuppression is also a risk factor for cervical cancer and CIN, for example patients on immunosuppressing drugs and those with AIDs.

Pathophysiology

The cervix is a tubular structure between the uterus and vagina and has undoubted importance in pregnancy. It is composed of stromal tissue which is lined by squamous epithelium in the vagina (ectocervix) and columnar epithelium within the cervical canal (endocervix). The endocervix contains many deep folds called crypts which are lined by columnar epithelium. The meeting of the two types of epithelial is called the squamocolumnar junction (SCJ) and this is usually at the ectocervix (Figure 14.1). The position of the SCJ varies throughout the reproductive years. In children it lies at the ectocervix, at puberty it extends outwards as the cervix enlarges and in adult life it returns to the ectocervix through the process of metaplasia, which is a physiological change from columnar epithelium to squamous epithelium. The transformation zone is an important area on the cervix which is defined as the area where the original SCJ was to the current SCJ and it includes areas of metaplasia. Occasionally, when the mucous columnar epithelium is covered by squamous epithelium there is retention of mucus – this is called a nabothian follicle (Figure 14.2). The transformation zone (TZ) is the site where premalignancy and malignancy develop.

HPV infection can persist in certain individuals, and for reasons unknown (possibly smoking) an oncogenic process can be triggered in the region of the TZ where metaplasia occurs. Integration of the viral DNA into the basal cells of the cervical epithelium in the TZ can lead to immortalization of the basal cells and rapid turnover of the basal cells within the epithelium. This disordered immaturity within the epithelium is called 'cervical intraepithelial neoplasia' and is truly an intraepithelial condition (cancer is diagnosed when this process breaks the basement membrane). CIN can be divided into low-grade (CIN 1) and high-grade disease (CIN 2 and 3).

Natural history of CIN

Regression and progression of CIN may occur. Spontaneous regression of low-grade disease is not uncommon and is likely to occur through the patient's own cell-mediated immunity. This is the argument for observational follow up in patients with low-grade abnormality. High-grade disease is less likely to regress spontaneously and requires treatment as there is a risk of progression to cancer. If left untreated, around 20 per cent of patients with high-grade abnormalities may develop cancer of the cervix. Reasons for this remain unclear but may include reduced host immunity, oncogenic (cancer causing) HPV types and smoking. There is a convincing link between CIN and cancer of the cervix as nearly all microscopic cancers of the cervix exist with CIN.

Cytology: cervical smears

Cells exfoliated from the cervix can be cytologically examined and act as a good screening test. Originally the 'Pap' smear was introduced by Papanicolou, where cells were removed from the cervix using a wooden spatula and placed on a glass slide and fixed. This was then examined by a cytologist for the immature squamous cells shed from the area of CIN. In the UK the 'Pap' smear has been superseded by liquid-based cytology where a small brush is used to sample cells from the transformation zone and the brush head placed in fixative (Figure 14.3). This is then spun down and then the cellular aspect of the specimen examined cytologically. Most cytological smears are normal and normal squamous cells are seen within the smear test. An abnormal smear can show cells in different degrees of maturity (dyskaryosis). Like CIN, cells can be classified as low grade (mild dyskaryosis and borderline change) or high grade (moderate and severe dyskaryosis) (Figure 14.4). There is some correlation between smear grade and the degrees of CIN on the cervix, but it is not totally reliable. Smears act as a means of referring patients to the colposcopy clinic for further assessment (see below under

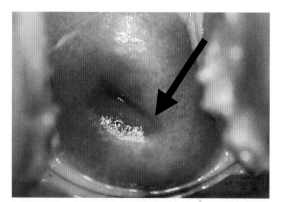

Figure 14.1 Normal cervix with transformation zone.

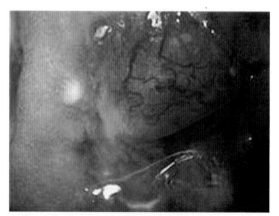

Figure 14.2 Normal cervix with nabothian follicle.

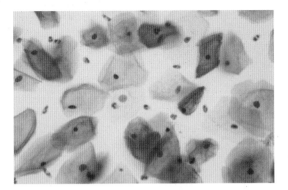

Figure 14.3   Liquid-based cytology – normal cytology.

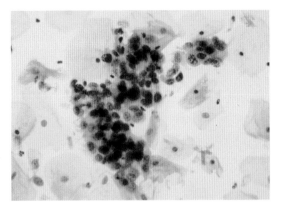

Figure 14.4   Liquid-based cytology – severe dyskaryosis.

Colposcopy). The sensitivity of the cervical smear in picking up women with CIN is around 70 per cent; however, as there is slow progression for most women with CIN to cancer, if a lesion is missed then this should be picked up on a subsequent smear.

Since 1988, the UK has offered population-based cervical screening for women. Women aged between 25 and 64 are invited every three to five years to take part in the screening programme and undergo a cervical smear with their GP. Most smears are negative and patients are placed on routine recall. Patients with high-grade smears (2 per cent) are referred urgently to colposcopy and patients with low-grade smear (4 per cent) have the smear repeated as minor changes may revert to normal. There is a large administrative need for the screening programme and the invitation for a smear is coordinated by the National Health Service Cervical Screening Programme (NHSCCP) which sends out computerized invitations to women. The coverage in the UK is around 85 per cent of the population. There has been a recent trend for a fall in uptake of smears in the 25–34 age group which is worrying. Reasons for this remain unclear, but may include ignorance and a lack of education about the importance of screening. Quality assurance is essential in the programme and there is a need for uniformly high standards in all aspects of the screening programme, including cytology, colposcopy and cervical pathology.

HPV vaccines

Cervical cancer and CIN is caused by HPV infection and in recent times HPV vaccines have been developed to prevent the primary infection with certain oncogenic HPV types (16, 18, 31, 33). Many countries have introduced a national programme of HPV vaccination with the sole aim of reducing death rates from cervical cancer through a prevention of HPV-related high-grade CIN. The evidence to date suggests that the vaccination is not only effective in preventing the development of high-grade CIN, but is safe to give. In the UK, a national programme of HPV vaccination to girls aged 12–13 started in 2009 to prevent HPV infection types 16 and 18. It will take many years to know if there will be a fall in the death rate. HPV vaccines are unlikely to eradicate cervical cancer in the long term as not all girls will be vaccinated. Other HPV types have been implicated in the pathogenesis of cervical cancer and the long-term benefits of the vaccine remain unknown.

Colposcopy

Colposcopy is the outpatient examination of the magnified cervix using a light source (Figure 14.5). It is used for both diagnosis and treatment. After a history and counselling, the woman undresses and places her legs in the semi-lithotomy position. A speculum is passed and the cervix examined with the light source under magnification (5 to 20×). Usually 5 per cent acetic acid and iodine are applied to the cervix and biopsies taken when necessary. Acetic acid causes nucleoproteins within cells to coagulate temporarily, therefore areas of increased cell turnover, for example in CIN will appear white at colposcopy (Figure 14.6). Areas of CIN lack the presence of intracellular glycogen and therefore stain yellow as opposed to the normal squamous epithelium which will stain brown when iodine is applied. CIN is a

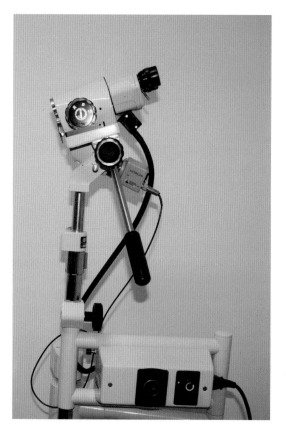

Figure 14.5   Colposcope.

pre-neoplastic process and the process of angiogenesis (new blood vessel formation) is apparent in CIN when viewed through the colposcope (Figure 14.7). The colposcopist will need to ask several questions including whether cervical cancer or CIN is present? If CIN is present, the colposcopist has to assess whether the appearances are low or high grade. The latter can be treated in the clinic on the same visit; the former can be monitored with a subsequent colposcopy and cytology six months later. A biopsy usually helps make the decision if unsure. All doctors and nurses carrying out colposcopy are required to undergo a period of training and examination to ensure high quality and standards of care are met. In addition, each colposcopy service undergoes a rigorous external quality assurance assessment every five years to ensure adequate standards are met.

Treatment of CIN

The aims of treatment are to effectively eradicate CIN, ensuring that post-treatment smears are negative,

while minimizing harm to the patient from the treatment. High-grade CIN requires treatment usually with excision or ablation. Low-grade CIN (CIN 1) may regress spontaneously in up to 60 per cent of cases, therefore close follow up with colposcopy and cytology six months after initial diagnosis is favoured as this avoids overtreating lesions that might have regressed. In the UK, the favoured method of treatment is loop diathermy (large loop excision of transformation zone, LLETZ). Under local anaesthetic, a diathermy wire loop is used to remove a portion of the cervix which includes the transformation zone with the area of CIN (Figure 14.8). CIN can develop deep within the cervical stroma and therefore excisional techniques need to be up to 10 mm deep. The procedure takes 15 minutes under local anaesthetic. The advantages of this excisional technique are that it is clinically effective (95 per cent of patients have negative smears at six months), cost-efficient (patient can be treated

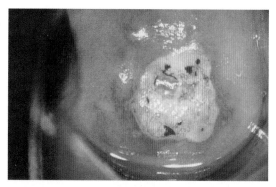

Figure 14.6   Cervix with acetic acid.

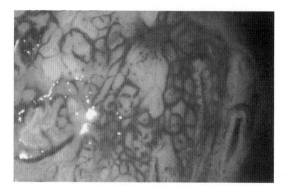

Figure 14.7   Cervix with cervical intraepithelial neoplasia (CIN) and new vessels.

at the first hospital visit) and it provides a specimen for pathological assessment (1 per cent of loop biopsies have an unsuspected microscopic cancer). The disadvantage relates to its potential impact on obstetric outcome. Small loops are likely to have no obstetric outcome; however, there is concern that if the loop excision of the cervix removes a large part of the cervix this might lead to preterm delivery through cervical weakening. This concern relates to young women who have not completed their family and where there may be the possibility of a second loop in the future (three loops is usually the maximal number of loops before a hysterectomy is considered). Recognizing the potential for overtreatment has been the main reason why women under 25 are not screened, as many lesions in this group of women are associated with HPV infection and might regress with observational follow up. Other options have been suggested for the treatment of CIN including cryotherapy, cold coagulation and cone biopsy.

Cryotherapy, where the cervix is frozen with liquid nitrogen as an outpatient, is sufficient treatment for low-grade CIN, but not effective enough for high-grade disease. The term 'cold coagulation' is a misnomer as the treatment involves placing a hot probe on the cervix in outpatients under local anaesthetic. It is a destructive treatment, is effective for both high- and low-grade CIN but does not provide a specimen. Cone biopsy involves cutting away a portion of the cervix under general anaesthetic and produces a specimen like a LLETZ. Its disadvantage relates to its need for a general anaesthetic and 5 per cent of patients may develop cervical stenosis or incompetence which has obstetric implications. It has been largely superseded by loop diathermy.

Patients who have undergone treatment require close follow up with regular cervical smears six monthly after treatment and then yearly for ten years, as they remain as a group at elevated risk of recurrent CIN and cervical cancer.

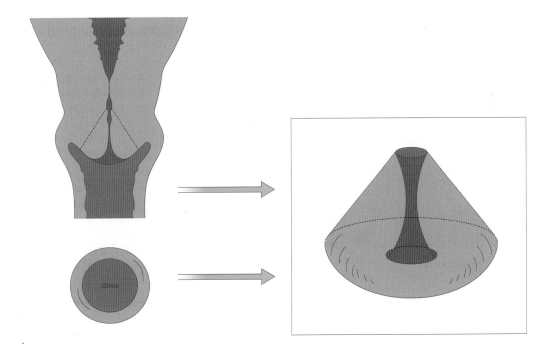

Figure 14.8   Large loop excision of transformation zone (LLETZ).

Malignant disease of the cervix

Clinical presentation

The clinical presentation is variable. Many patients are asymptomatic as the cancer has been diagnosed as an incidental finding after a loop biopsy of the cervix for pre-invasive disease. This is not uncommon as microscopic cervical cancers are difficult to identify colposcopically and are only identified on subsequent histological examination. Most cervical cancers, however, are friable, vascular masses on the cervix and are likely to produce a number of complaints including post-coital bleeding, intermenstrual bleeding, post-menopausal bleeding and blood-stained vaginal discharge (Figure 14.9). Any woman with these symptoms therefore should undergo a full history and abdominal pelvic examination, including visualization of the cervix. In advanced disease (stages 3–4), patients may experience a number of distressing symptoms including pain (malignant infiltration of the spinal cord), incontinence (due to vesicovaginal fistulae), anaemia (from chronic vaginal bleeding) and renal failure (from ureteric blockage).

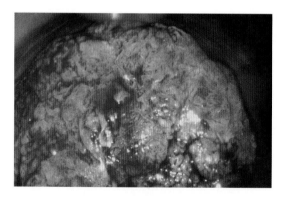

Figure 14.9   Cervical cancer.

Initial clinical assessment of patients may be unrevealing as the disease is often locally not visible, even in advanced disease. A pelvic and speculum examination usually clinches the diagnosis as there is often a cervical mass which bleeds on contact and if advanced disease, a hardness and fixity of the tissues. A biopsy in the outpatient should be taken. Very occasionally, the diagnosis can be missed as some tumours are endophytic rather than exophytic and therefore less clinically revealing. The clinician therefore needs to retain a level of clinical suspicion in the presence of unexplained symptoms and investigate patients with persistent problems.

Pathophysiology

The majority (70 per cent) of cervical cancers are squamous cell carcinomas with adenocarcinomas making up most of the remainder. In the developed world, with screening programmes, there has been a relative fall in the numbers of squamous tumours and a relative rise in the incidence of adenocarcinomas. In the UK, 30 per cent of tumours are adenocarcinomas and are less likely to be picked up on cervical screening. The tumours are locally infiltrative in the pelvic area, but also spread via lymphatics and in the late stages via blood vessels. The tumour can grow through the cervix to reach the parametria (anatomical area lateral to the cervix), bladder, vagina and rectum. Metastases can occur therefore in pelvic (iliac and obturator) and para-aortic nodes and, in the later stages, liver and lungs.

Investigation and the importance of staging

Assessing the stage of the disease is crucial for giving the patient an idea of prognosis and planning treatment. Staging for cervical cancer is given in Table 14.1. Patients are staged according to the system introduced by the International Federation of Obstetricians and Gynaecologists (FIGO). A biopsy is crucial to confirm malignancy and assess the tumour type. An MR scan of the abdomen and pelvis will assess the local spread of the disease in the cervix and will detect enlarged lymph nodes in the pelvis area. A chest x-ray is vital to exclude lung metastases. An examination under anaesthetic may be helpful when, despite the above tests, the clinician is still unclear whether the tumour is operable. Doing a rectovaginal examination under anaesthetic can give crucial information on the tumour including size of disease, fixity and vaginal involvement, and a cystoscopy can help eliminate bladder involvement. Small mobile tumours favour a surgical approach, whereas larger fixed tumours favour the use of radiotherapy. The FIGO staging includes an intravenous urogram to ensure the integrity of the ureters; however, this is not

Table 14.1   Staging and prognosis of cervical cancer (FIGO)

Stage	Description	Five-year survival rate (%)
1	**Carcinoma confined to the cervix** (corpus extension should be disregarded) 1a: Invasive cancer identified only microscopically. All gross lesions, even with superficial invasion, are stage 1b cancers. Depth of measured stromal invasion should not be greater than 5 mm and no wider than 7 mm 1a1: Measured invasion no greater than 3 mm in depth and no wider than 7 mm 1a2: Measured depth of invasion greater than 3 mm and no greater than 5 mm and no wider than 7 mm 1b: Clinical lesions confined to the cervix or preclinical lesions greater than 1a 1b1: Clinical lesions no greater than 4 cm in size 1b2: Clinical lesions greater than 4 cm in size	83
2	**Carcinoma extending beyond the cervix and involving the vagina** (but not the lower third) and/or infiltrating the parametrium (but not reaching the pelvic sidewall) 2a: Carcinoma has involved the vagina 2b: Carcinoma has infiltrated the parametrium	65
3	**Carcinoma involving the lower third of the vagina and/or extending to the pelvic sidewall** (there is no free space between the tumour and the pelvic sidewall) 3a: Carcinoma involving the lower third of the vagina 3b: Carcinoma extending to the pelvic wall and/or hydronephrosis or non-functioning kidney due to ureteric obstruction caused by tumour	36
4	4a: Carcinoma involving the mucosa of the bladder or rectum and/or extending beyond the true pelvis 4b: Spread to distant organs	10

standard practice in the developed world where MRI has superseded such tests. The staging of the disease is based on clinical findings unlike other gynaecological tumours where there is a reliance on surgery and pathology to give the ultimate stage. The reasons for this are that radiotherapy is used in advanced disease and it still remains possible to stage patients in the developing world where most of the disease occurs.

Treatment

Treatment is given depending on the stage of the disease and the age and fitness of the patient. Ideally, all cancer patients should be discussed within the context of a multidisciplinary team of doctors (surgeons, radiotherapists, radiologists and pathologists) and nurses, so that the most appropriate treatment can be offered to the patient. The fitness of the patient is crucial before embarking on treatment as radical surgery may not be appropriate in an unfit patient.

Preclinical lesions: stage 1a

These microscopic tumours have a low volume of cancer and are usually picked up as incidental findings after loop diathermy. Small lesions need to have a clear margin of excision, but also the pre-invasive disease (CIN) that invariably coexists must also be completely excised as occasionally the cancer can be multifocal. If the pre-invasive disease is not completely excised then a repeat loop biopsy or knife cone biopsy must be carried out. This treatment enables fertility to be preserved and a hysterectomy is not necessary.

Clinical invasive cervical carcinoma: stages 1b–4

The tumour volumes are much greater in patients with stage 1a disease and therefore fertility-preserving treatment for this group of patients is usually not an option. When the disease is confined to the cervix (stage 1b), then radical hysterectomy and pelvic node dissection (Wertheim's hysterectomy) should be considered in pre-menopausal patients. It is important to remember that in early stage 1b disease pelvic radiotherapy has similar success rates as surgery and therefore this treatment can be considered in pre-menopausal patients who are too overweight for radical surgery or who are anaesthetically unfit. The benefits of surgery are discussed in the following section (Surgery). Radiotherapy may be the treatment of choice in post-menopausal patients with early stage 1b disease as the urological complication rates following radical surgery are higher due to tissue fragility. Occasionally, patients with small volume cancers that are just outside the stage of 1a2 but fall into stage 1b1 on measurement may be suitable for fertility sparing treatment (radical trachelectomy). As the disease affects young women then this might be appropriate if a patient has not started her family. The radical trachelectomy operation involves removing 80 per cent of the cervix and parametrial tissues together with resection of the pelvic lymph nodes. Problems can occur with follow up (no cervix to view) and the mid-trimester miscarriage rate can be as high as 40 per cent. Counselling these patients on the risks/benefits of this operation is paramount.

When the disease is beyond the cervix (stages 2–4 disease) then radiotherapy (with or without chemotherapy) becomes the optimal treatment. Surgery in isolation is problematic as complications can occur (severe haemorrhage) and also achieving clearance of the tumour is unlikely. Incomplete excision of cancer from surgery requires adjuvant postoperative radiotherapy and the combined treatments can lead to high complication rates. As an oncological rule it is not wise to cut through cancer.

Surgery

The standard surgical operation for stage 1b tumours is a radical hysterectomy and pelvic lymph node dissection. This involves removal of the cervix, upper third of the vagina, uterus and the parametrial tissue. Pelvic lymph node removal includes the obturator, internal and external iliac nodes. The ovaries in pre-menopausal women can be spared. There is higher morbidity of this procedure over the standard total abdominal hysterectomy. Bladder dysfunction (atony), sexual dysfunction (due to vaginal shortening) and lymphoedema (due to removal of the pelvic lymph nodes) are not uncommon. An atonic bladder is frequent in the immediate postoperative period due to neuronal damage from the surgery, and intermittent self-catheterization may be required until the bladder tone returns. Lymphoedema is variable and is described by patients as a wooden, heavy feeling to the legs with swelling and reduced mobility. Management includes leg elevation, good skin care (e.g. avoid shaving) massage and occasionally compression stockings. Despite these potential problems, surgery is the preferred treatment as the cure rate is high, ovarian tissue can be preserved and the patient avoids the complications of radiotherapy (see below).

Radiotherapy

The aim of radiotherapy is to deliver a lethal dose of radiation to the tumour and minimize damage to the surrounding tissues. Treatment is overseen by a radiotherapist and team. Treatment is delivered in two ways: external beam radiotherapy (as teletherapy) and internal radiotherapy (brachytherapy). In external beam radiotherapy, the source of the radiation is from a machine called a linear accelerator, and radiation is delivered to the pelvis a distance from the patient (Figure 14.10). The dose of radiotherapy is carefully calculated according to the patient and the tumour, and is usually administered as 45 Gy in total. This is given in several treatments or 'fractions' as an outpatient over 4 weeks. Although this treatment is given daily, the time of each fraction is no more than 10 minutes. Brachytherapy is a radiotherapy technique where the radiation is delivered internally to the patient. The source of the radiation is usually selenium and patients usually have to undergo an examination under anaesthetic to insert the rods into the uterus. These rods are then attached to the radiotherapy source; the patient receives this internal treatment in isolation to protect the staff. Brachytherapy delivers a high dose of radiation to the tumour source and its harmful effects on the bladder and bowel are minimized as its effects are targeted only 5 mm from the rod.

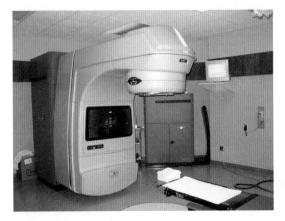

Figure 14.10   Linear accelerator.

Patients frequently suffer lethargy with treatment and may experience both bowel and bladder urgency, which is due to the initial inflammatory effects of the radiation. Skin erythema-like sunburn is not uncommon. Symptomatic treatment is usually required, such as anti-inflammatory creams for skin. Around 5 per cent of patients experience a serious side effect that might interrupt treatment, for example bowel perforation. There are many long-term complications of radiotherapy which affect a minority of patients but which do have a significant impact on patients' quality of life. The initial inflammatory process is replaced by fibrosis in the long term. Vaginal stenosis can cause sexual pain, bladder damage can lead to cystitis-like symptoms, haematuria and bowel damage lead to malabsorption and mucous diarrhoea. None of these complications can be managed easily. Patients who are pre-menopausal will undergo a radiotherapy-induced menopause as the ovaries are very sensitive to small doses of irradiation.

Chemotherapy (cisplatin) is ideally given in conjunction with the radiotherapy as this combination increases cure rates more than when radiotherapy is used in isolation. It probably works by enhancing the effects of radiotherapy and might also address micrometastases which are outside the radiotherapy field.

Palliative treatment

When it is not possible to offer curative treatment then palliation of symptoms becomes important and early involvement of the palliative care team is essential for symptom control. The disease can be greatly hidden from family and friends even in the late stages of the disease; patients may be experiencing a number of symptoms from local infiltration of the pelvis by the cancer. Malignant pain, recto- and/or vesicovaginal fistulae and bleeding may occur. Distant spread is often a very late stage of the disease. Radiotherapy may be considered with a palliative intent, for example a one-off treatment with radiotherapy may be used for symptomatic bone metastases.

Key Points

- Cervical cancer is a disease commonly affecting women in the developing world. Most women never see a health professional in their life and die from their disease in their community.

- Population-based cervical screening of adult women has prevented 70 per cent of cases of cervical cancer developing in the UK. HPV vaccination of children in schools is likely to reduce rates further, but this will take many years to be of benefit.

- All patient with symptoms of cervical cancer, e.g. post-coital bleeding, intermenstrual bleeding should have a full pelvic examination.

CHAPTER 15

CONDITIONS AFFECTING THE VAGINA AND VULVA

OVERVIEW

Vulval problems are common, misdiagnosed and often poorly managed by health professionals. It is essential that a good history and clinical examination is carried out supplemented by any relevant investigations. Chronic vulval disease has a major impact on the patient's life and different components of the problem may need addressing, such as sexual dysfunction and chronic pain management. A team approach may be necessary using gynaecologists, dermatologists and genitourinary medicine physicians. Many vulval clinics have been set up in hospitals in the spirit of team working and bringing different skills together to tackle chronic vulval problems.

Introduction

The vulva is the term used to describe the external female genitalia – the sexual organs. It includes the labia majora and minor, clitoris and fourchette (see Figure 15.1). The vulval vestibule is defined anatomically as the area between the lower end of the vaginal canal at the hymenal ring and the labia minora. The different anatomical areas of the external genitalia have different histological characteristics and embryological origins. Both the labia minora and majora are covered with keratinized, pigmented, squamous epithelium. The labia majora are two large folds of adipose tissue covered by skin containing hair follicles, sebaceous and sweat glands. In contrast, the labia minora are devoid of adipose tissue and hair follicles, but contain sebaceous follicles. The normal vulval vestibule is covered with non-keratinized, non-pigmented squamous epithelium and is devoid of skin adnexa. Within the vulval vestibule are the ducts of the minor vestibular glands, the periurethral glands of Skene, the urethral meatus and the ducts of the Bartholin's glands. The Bartholin's glands (major vestibular glands) are the major glands of the vestibule and lie deep within the perineum. Both the major and the minor vestibular glands contain mucous-secreting acini with ducts lined by transitional epithelium. The ducts of the Bartholin's glands exit at the introitus just above the fourchette at approximately five and seven o'clock on the perineum and those of the minor vestibular glands are distributed throughout the vulval vestibule. The vagina and vulva are commonly known as the lower genital tract with the vagina leading to the upper genital tract (uterus, cervix, tubes and ovaries).

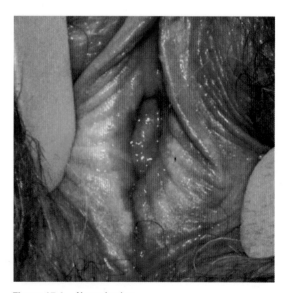

Figure 15.1　Normal vulva.

The vagina has is a tubular structure but has anterior and posterior walls which lie in opposition.

Vulval skin has different physiological properties when compared to other regions of the body such as the forearm. Transepidermal water loss is twice the amount in vulval skin compared to forearm skin. This suggests that the stratum corneum, the protective layer of vulval skin, functions poorly as a skin barrier when compared to other skin areas and may explain why vulval skin is more prone to irritancy.

Assessment

A full history and clinical examination (with optional vaginal swabs and biopsies) are essential to make the diagnosis. Vulval skin is an extension of general skin surfaces and it is important in the history to ask about general skin problems as this might point towards the diagnosis, for example psoriasis or eczema can synchronously affect the vulva and the limbs. The history should focus on the presenting complaint. It is important to discuss current methods of skin care (e.g. use of scented products which can aggravate symptoms), which topical treatments are being used (e.g. some creams such as antifungals can aggravate the problem) and the impact of the symptoms on sexual functioning. The clinical examination should include all skin surfaces and the vulval area should be examined systematically with a good light source.

Vulval pruritus, pain and superficial dyspareunia are common symptoms and Table 15.1 illustrates the differential diagnoses of different symptoms, although this is not an exhaustive list. Confusingly for the clinician, most patients have more than one symptom.

After a full history and clinical examination, it should be possible to make a provisional diagnosis. Sometimes it is necessary to carry out some swabs

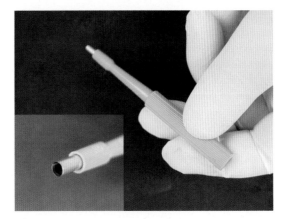

Figure 15.2   Keyes punch biopsy.

and a biopsy for confirmation. Microbiological swabs may be indicated to exclude infection as a cause of vulval symptoms (e.g. candida and *Trichomonas vaginalis* can cause vulval itching, herpes simplex may cause vulval ulcers). When there is a lesion on the vulva and the diagnosis is unclear, then an outpatient vulval biopsy is helpful. The Keyes punch biopsy is a 4-mm sample of skin that can be taken under local anaesthetic in the clinic (Figure 15.2). A pathology sample allows an accurate diagnosis to be made and the correct treatment to be instigated. Biopsies should be carried out when there is a pigmented lesion, a raised or indurated area and a persistent ulcer.

Treatment principles

Treatment should be given based on a correct diagnosis and empirical treatment should be discouraged because of the potential side effects of treatment. Good skin care of the vulva is essential, with an avoidance of scented and over-the-counter products as these can

Table 15.1   Differential diagnosis of vulval complaints

Vulval pruritus	Vulval pain	Superficial dyspareunia
Infections, e.g. candidiasis, *Trichomonas vaginalis*	Infections, e.g. candidiasis	Skin conditions, e.g. lichen sclerosus (causes vulval splitting)
Skin conditions, e.g. lichen sclerosis, eczema, VIN	Skin conditions, e.g. lichen sclerosis, eczema, VIN	Vulvodynia
Contact dermatitis	Vulvodynia	Vulval fissures
		Skin bridges of the vulva

produce unnecessary irritancy on the skin. Emollients are bland scent-free topical products that can soothe and rehydrate the skin and can be used liberally, for example aqueous cream. When prescribing cream, for example steroid ointments, it is important to be clear to patients how much, when and where to apply the treatment. Patients value showing them the application of the ointments or creams in the clinic. Dosage is important particularly when prescribing steroids. One finger-tip-unit of cream or ointment is from the last crease in the index finger to the tip and equates to 0.5 g. A 30-g tube when used twice a day therefore should last for a month.

Benign conditions

Some of the common conditions are discussed below.

Lichen sclerosis

Lichen sclerosis is a destructive inflammatory skin condition which affects mainly the anogenital area of women. It is believed to affect 1 in 300 women and the cause is believed to be autoimmune. Many patients have other autoimmune conditions, such as thyroid disease and pernicious anaemia. The destructive nature of the condition is due to underlying inflammation in the subdermal layers of the skin which results in hyalinization of the skin. This leads to a fragility and white 'parchment paper' appearance of the skin and loss of vulval anatomy (Figure 15.3). The condition can involve the foreskin of men to produce a phimosis. Fifteen per cent of patients have evidence of lichen sclerosis elsewhere on the body. The main symptoms on the vulva is itching and subsequent soreness of the vulva, usually due to scratching. Splitting of the skin is common and frequently occurs at the posterior fourchette which can lead to superficial dyspareunia. On examination of the skin, whitening, fissuring and loss of anatomy are common in long-standing cases, but appearances can be subtle in early stage disease. A biopsy can confirm the diagnosis and treatment is a combination of good skin care and strong steroid ointments, such as Dermovate. Lichen sclerosis is associated with vulval cancer, but is not a cause. Many women with vulval cancer have lichen sclerosis at the time of diagnosis and it is estimated that there is a low risk of cancer developing in a women with lichen sclerosis (around 3–5 per cent).

Vulvodynia

Vulvodynia describes a group of women with vulval discomfort, most often described as a burning pain, occurring in the absence of skin disease or infection. It is akin to a neuropathic pain syndrome. Patients can be further classified by the anatomical site of the pain (e.g. generalized, localized and clitoral) and also by whether pain is provoked or unprovoked. Patients have a spectrum of disease. Some patients have continuous burning, some have sexual pain only and some have both. The cause is not known. Clinical examination is normal, although some patient have touch sensitivity – so-called allodynia. This is the phenomenon when there is reprogramming of the nerve endings from touch to pain. The diagnosis is clinical and treatments can vary. Patients with sexual pain may require psychosexual counselling and vulval desensitization (e.g. massage and the use of vaginal trainers), whereas patients with unprovoked pain may benefit from drugs, such as the tricyclic antidepressants or the anticonvulsants, which are commonly used in many chronic pain conditions.

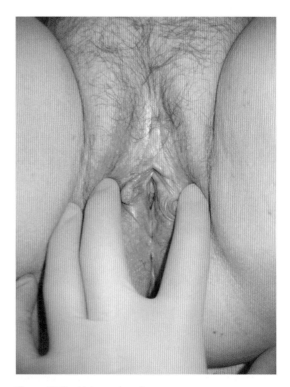

Figure 15.3   Lichen sclerosis.

Genital herpes simplex

Genital herpes simplex is the most common cause of reported vulval ulceration seen within departments of genitourinary medicine in the UK. Two serotypes (types 1 and 2) are responsible for both oral and genital ulceration with increasing numbers of genital infections being caused by type 1. The clinical presentation is variable with either a primary or secondary infection. The typical history of herpetic illness is irritation or paraesthesia at the site of the lesion before the appearance of painful papules. These form vesicles that erode to give superficial erosions that either heal or form ulcers. The ulcers are often multiple, shallow-based, flat and small. There is often an erythematous halo around the ulcers and surrounding oedema. With time, crusting and healing of the lesion occurs and the whole episode is completed on average within a week. Following an attack, the skin heals without scarring. Primary infections can be associated with a severe attack and viraemic symptoms. Recurrent infections occur in 50 per cent of patients and tend to be less severe.

In the acute phase, antiviral agents (acyclovir 200 mg orally five times per day for 5 days) will reduce the length of viral shedding and shorten the healing time in the primary attack. In recurrent herpes, suppression therapy should be considered with long-term acyclovir. Referral to a genitourinary medicine department may be considered for opportunistic screening and counselling, as for some the psychosexual impact of the diagnosis is considerable. There are many other causes of vulval ulcers such as trauma, Behçet's syndrome, Crohn's disease and fixed drug eruptions.

Benign cysts of the vulva

Bartholin's cysts, Skene gland cysts and mucous inclusion cysts can affect the vulval area and cause a lump with or without vulval discomfort. If they do not cause the patient any problem, they can be either monitored or excised. A Bartholin's cyst is the most common type of cyst and develops in the region of the Bartholin's gland (Figure 15.4). The Bartholin's gland has a long duct which, when blocked, causes fluid to build up and eventually a cyst. It is not uncommon for these cysts to get infected and cause a Bartholin's abscess which usually presents acutely and may require incision and drainage. Marsupialization of the cyst is

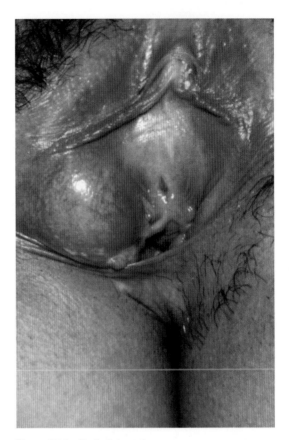

Figure 15.4   Bartholin's cyst.

the term used when the internal aspect of the cyst is sutured to the outside of the cyst to create a window so that the cyst does not reform. Marsupialization of Bartholin's cysts is usually elective.

Vulval intraepithelial neoplasia

Vulval intraepitheial neoplasia (VIN) is a premalignant skin condition which is increasing in incidence. VIN can be either associated with human papilloma viruses (HPV) or with lichen sclerosis. HPV-associated VIN can occur in pre-menopausal women and lichen sclerosis-associated HPV in older, often post-menopausal women. The clinical presentation is variable with either pain and/or pruritus. On clinical examination, patients may have a variety of findings from indurated, pigmented lesions to eroded red areas on the labia (Figure 15.5). A biopsy is essential for diagnosis and it is important to exclude invasive disease that might coexist.

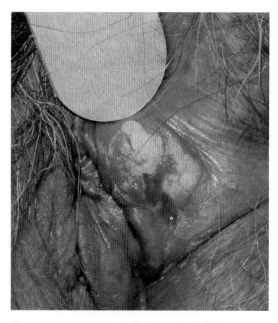

Figure 15.5   Vulval intraepithelial neoplasia (VIN).

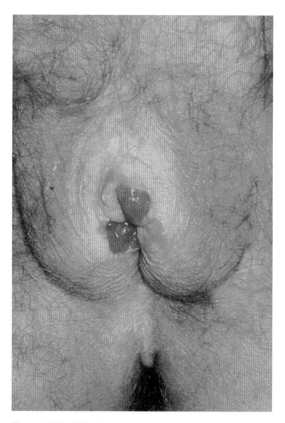

Figure 15.6   Vulval cancer.

Treatment depends on the patient's symptoms and the nature of the lesion. Options include surgical excision of the area, laser treatment, immunomodulating creams or observational follow up. Each treatment method has its advantages and disadvantages. Surgery for example can quickly remove localized areas, but recurrence rates are high (up to 40 per cent) and removal of skin can be disfiguring if the disease is near the clitorus. Immunomodulating creams (e.g. imiquimod) can avoid potentially disfiguring surgery but the response rates are around 60 per cent and the cream can cause significant skin burning.

Vulval cancers

Vulval cancer is uncommon, with an incidence of ten cases per 100 000 women. There are around 1000 newly diagnosed cases a year in the UK. These are skin tumours of the vulva and are divided into HPV-associated (usually younger patients) and non-HPV (usually older patients) cancers. The latter group may have their cancer associated with VIN and lichen sclerosis.

Clinical presentation

Vulval cancers usually present with vulval symptoms. Patients may present with a lump (noticed when washing), vulval pain (some tumours are ulcerating) and post-menopausal bleeding (some tumours bleed on touch). Some patients are frequently unaware of vulval cancer. While most tumours are small on examination, it is surprising how large some tumours can be on initial presentation.

The tumours are usually clinically obvious and are often cauliflower-type growths on the vulva (Figure 15.6). Some tumours, however, can ulcerate and some may produce a subtle skin thickening. The most common sites are the labia majora and clitoris and the tumours may be uni- or multifocal so it is important to examine the patient thoroughly (include the anal area, vagina and cervix). Vulval cancer spreads regionally to the groin nodes (inguinal and femoral) and palpation of these nodes is important to exclude clinically obvious malignant nodes. Patients should also have the cervix inspected to make sure that there is no involvement by cancer or cervical intraepithelial neoplasia (CIN).

Pathophysiology

Most vulval cancers are squamous cell cancers of the skin. The lymphatic drainage of the vulva (and the lower third of the vagina) is to the inguinal and femoral lymph nodes and this is the first place to which the tumour metastasizes. Beyond this, the tumour can spread up the lymphatic chain and finally to the liver and lungs at a late stage. Rarely vulval melanoma can develop and present with ulcerated and/or pigmented lesions. Treatment is by surgical excision of the primary site only. Prognosis is poor and related to the depth of invasion.

Investigation and the importance of staging

A biopsy is essential for diagnosis and a chest x-ray is useful to exclude obvious lung metastases. Staging of the cancer is essential for prognostic information and planning adjuvant treatment (Table 15.2). Poor prognostic factors include large (greater than 4 cm) primary tumours, sphincter involvement and metastases to the groin nodes.

Treatment

As the tumours are locally invasive and frequently symptomatic, then surgery is the best approach. Surgery involves excision of the primary site and removal of the groin lymph nodes. Removal of the primary tumour requires a wide and deep excision to give clear surgical margins of usually 1–2 cm (radical wide local excision). With extensive disease, the whole vulva may need removal (radical vulvectomy). Incomplete surgical margins are a problem as they can lead to local recurrences at the site of surgery. Around 30 per cent of patients suitable for surgery have groin node metastases and therefore the tumour excision is usually combined with a unilateral or bilateral inguinofemoral lymphadenectomy. If the nodes are positive, then postoperative radiotherapy is given to treat any residual disease in the groin. The surgery has many problems for patients as it can be disfiguring and frequently results in psychosexual issues. Seventy per cent of patients undergoing a groin node dissection have negative nodes, but still run the risk of lymphoedema and lymphocyst formation. Patients with lymphoedema describe a heavy, 'wooden', sometimes painful feeling in the legs as a result of retention of lymph fluid. This can cause reduced mobility and problems wearing shoes. Management involves leg elevation, good skin care, massage of the limbs and, in severe cases, support stockings. The sentinel lymph node (SLN) procedure may replace groin node dissection in the future where the SLN (the first lymph node to be involved with metastases) is identified and removed in isolation. If this node is negative, the patient is followed up and if positive, radiotherapy is given. Further trials are needed to determine whether this can be safely used as an established technique.

Advanced disease (stages 3 and 4) is difficult as patients often die from disease. Patients are treated

Table 15.2 Staging and prognosis of vulval cancer (FIGO 2009)

Stage	Description	5-year survival rate (%)
1	1a: Confined to vulva and/or perineum, 2 cm or less maximum diameter. Groin nodes not palpable. Stromal invasion no greater than 1 mm 1b: As for 1a but stromal invasion <1 mm	93
2	Confined to vulva and/or perineum, more than 2 cm maximum diameter. Groin nodes not palpable	80
3	Extends beyond the vulva, vagina, lower urethra or anus; or unilateral regional lymph node metastasis	35
4	4a: Involves the mucosa of rectum or bladder upper urethra; or pelvic bone; and/or bilateral regional lymph node metastases 4b: Any distant metastasis including pelvic lymph nodes	10

with combinations of surgery (to remove malignant nodes), radiotherapy and chemotherapy. This is a difficult treatment as patients are often elderly and radiotherapy to the vulval skin frequently produces pain through skin desquamation. Palliative care input therefore is important at an early stage.

Vaginal disease

The main vaginal problem is infection which is covered in Chapter 6, Genital infections in gynaecology. Bacterial (bacterial vaginosis), fungal (*Candida albicans*) and protozoal (*Trichomonas vaginalis*) infections can produce vaginal inflammation and discharge. Microbiological swabs will confirm the diagnosis and the symptoms should soon resolve. Few skin conditions affect the vagina. Worthy of mention is erosive lichen planus of the vagina which is an autoimmune inflammatory skin condition that causes vaginal pain, inflammation and if untreated vaginal stenosis. Treatment is usually with vaginal trainers (to stretch the narrowing) and intravaginal steroids. Conditions affecting the vulva, such as lichen sclerosis and eczema, do not affect the vagina.

Intraepithelial neoplasia can affect the genital tract (CIN and VIN) as discussed above and in Chapter 14, Premalignant and malignant disease of the cervix. The vaginal area can also be affected (called vaginal intraepithelial neoplasia, VAIN). This is usually as a result of extension of CIN from the cervix. VAIN is asymptomatic. Treatment can involve cauterization, surgical excision, radiotherapy and observational follow up depending on the patient, grade of disease and size of the lesion. VAIN assessment and treatment can be complicated and is best managed by specialist teams. There is a risk of vaginal cancer in untreated patients, but this risk remains unclear.

Vaginal cancer

This is a rare cancer that accounts for around 250 new cases a year. The cause remains unknown, although the risk factors are likely to be similar to cervical cancer (see Chapter14, Premalignant and malignant

disease of the cervix). The disease frequently presents at an advanced stage in the absence of symptoms with early disease (Table 15.3). When the disease becomes symptomatic vaginal bleeding and discharge are the presenting features. Pain may be present if the disease has extended beyond the vaginal area and infiltrated pelvic nerves. The diagnosis is with a vaginal biopsy and the investigation of patients is the same as for cervical cancer. Surgery is rarely an option as the disease is advanced and radiotherapy and chemotherapy are usually first-line treatments. Disease progression is usually local and, in the advanced stages of the disease, patients may develop symptoms that are difficult to palliate, such as rectovaginal and vesicovaginal fistulae.

Table 15.3   FIGO staging and prognosis of vaginal cancer

Stage	Description	5-year survival rate (%)
1	Invasive carcinoma confined to vaginal mucosa	89
2	Subvaginal infiltration not extending to pelvic wall	60
3	Extends to pelvic wall	35
4	4a: Involves mucosa of bladder or rectum 4b: Spread beyond the pelvis	10

Key Points

- All patients with vulval symptoms require a detailed history and clinical examination.

- If the diagnosis is not clear, then a biopsy and vaginal swabs can be helpful. Giving the patient information on bland hygiene measures and emollients can help for symptomatic improvement. Any pigmented, raised lesion should be biopsied.

- In the presence of symptoms and a normal examination, think of vulvodynia.

- For difficult patients, a vulval clinic might be an appropriate setting for patients to be reviewed.

OVERVIEW

Urogynaecological conditions include urinary incontinence, voiding difficulties, prolapse (see also Chapter 17, Pelvic organ prolapse), frequency and urgency, urinary tract infection and urinary fistulae. Increasingly, it is recognized that the pelvic floor is one structure and this has led to increased understanding of faecal incontinence and to improvements in its treatment.

Clinical conditions

Introduction

Urinary incontinence is defined as the involuntary loss of urine that is objectively demonstrable and is a social or hygienic problem. It is increasingly prevalent as the ageing population expands. It affects an individual's physical, psychological and social well-being and is associated with a significant reduction in quality of life. The prevalence increases with age, with approximately 5 per cent of women between 15 and 44 years of age being affected, rising to 10 per cent of those aged between 45 and 64 years, and approximately 20 per cent of those older than 65 years. It is even higher in women who are institutionalized and may affect up to 40 per cent of those in residential nursing homes.

Common symptoms associated with incontinence

- Stress incontinence is a symptom and a sign and means loss of urine on physical effort. It is not a diagnosis.
- Urgency means a sudden desire to void.
- Urge incontinence is an involuntary loss of urine associated with a strong desire to void.
- Overflow incontinence occurs without any detrusor activity when the bladder is overdistended.
- Frequency is defined as the passing of urine seven or more times a day, or being awoken from sleep more than once a night to void.

Urinary incontinence is classified according to pathophysiological concepts rather than symptomatology, but the following definitions of symptoms are commonly used.

In addition, women may also have complaints of prolapse, sexual dysfunction due to leakage and coexisting anal incontinence. Haematuria in the absence of infection requires prompt urological referral.

Urethral causes

Urodynamic stress incontinence

Urodynamic stress incontinence (USI), previously called genuine stress incontinence, is noted during filling cystometry, and is defined as the involuntary leakage of urine during increased abdominal pressure in the absence of a detrusor contraction.

Symptoms

Stress incontinence is the usual symptom, but urgency, frequency and urge incontinence may be present. There may also be an awareness of prolapse. On clinical examination, stress incontinence may be demonstrated when the patient coughs. Vaginal examination should assess for prolapse and, in particular, the vaginal capacity and the woman's ability to elevate the bladder neck, as this may alter management. It is not unusual to find a cystourethrocele in women with stress incontinence, but there is no causal relationship.

Urodynamic studies will define the cause of incontinence and are particularly important when

Understanding the pathophysiology

The likely causes of USI are as follows:

- Abnormal descent of the bladder neck and proximal urethra, so there is failure of equal transmission of intra-abdominal pressure to the proximal urethra, leading to reversal of the normal pressure gradient between the bladder and urethra, with a resultant negative urethral closure pressure.

- An intraurethral pressure which at rest is lower than the intravesical pressure; this may be due to urethral scarring as a result of surgery or radiotherapy. It also occurs in older women due to oestrogen deficiency.

- Laxity of suburethral support normally provided by the vaginal wall, endopelvic fascia, arcus tendineus fascia and levator ani muscles acting as a single unit results in ineffective compression during physical stress and consequent incontinence (Figure 16.1).

there has been a previous, unsuccessful continence operation or if the symptomatology is complex (these factors are covered later in this chapter).

The aetiology of USI is thought to be related to a number of factors:

- Damage to the nerve supply of the pelvic floor and urethral sphincter caused by childbirth leads to progressive changes in these structures, resulting in altered function. In addition, mechanical trauma to the pelvic floor musculature and endopelvic fascia and ligaments occurs as a consequence of vaginal delivery. Prolonged second stage, large babies and instrumental deliveries cause the most damage.

- Menopause and associated tissue atrophy may also cause damage to the pelvic floor.

- A congenital cause may be inferred, as some nulliparous women suffer from incontinence. This may be due to altered connective tissue, particularly collagen. Stress incontinence is much less common in black women and differences in connective tissue are thought to be responsible.

- Chronic causes, such as obesity and chronic obstructive pulmonary disease, raise interabdominal pressure, and constipation and associated straining may also result in problems.

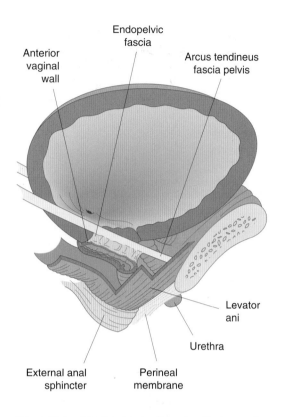

Figure 16.1   Diagram showing the suburethral support mechanism.

Detrusor overactivity

Detrusor overactivity, previously called detrusor instability, is a urodynamic observation characterized by involuntary detrusor contractions during the filling phase which may be spontaneous or provoked.

Understanding the pathophysiology

Detrusor overactivity

The pathophysiology of detrusor overactivity is poorly understood and the aetiological factors require substantiation. Poor toilet habit training and psychological factors have been implicated. More recently, there have been suggestions that urinary tract infection may be a trigger, but further research is required.

The largest group of women with this condition have an idiopathic variety which is more prevalent after the menopause. Childhood enuresis increases the likelihood of developing symptoms of overactivity.

Neuropathy appears to be the most substantiated factor. Incontinence surgery, outflow obstruction and smoking are also associated with detrusor overactivity.

The combination of symptoms of urgency, frequency and nocturia is termed the overactive bladder (OAB) syndrome with (OAB wet) or without (OAB dry) urgency incontinence, in the absence of urinary tract infection or other obvious pathology. Urgency is the complaint of a sudden, compelling desire to void which is difficult to defer. This group of symptoms has a much more deleterious effect on quality of life than stress incontinence. Women with OAB are more restricted and often map their journeys around the location of toileting facilities.

Classification of incontinence

Urethral causes

- Urethral sphincter incompetence (urodynamic stress incontinence)
- Detrusor overactivity or the unstable bladder – this is either neurogenic or non-neurogenic
- Retention with overflow
- Congenital causes
- Miscellaneous
- Extraurethral causes
- Congenital causes
- Fistula

Examination

Any masses that cause compression of the bladder must be excluded and prolapse must be examined for, as this may cause some of the symptoms. If there is vaginal atrophy, this may also cause some urgency and frequency. Observation of involuntary loss of urine from the urethra, synchronous with coughing, may suggest stress incontinence.

Observation of urine leakage through channels other than the urethra may suggest a congenital anomaly or fistula.

Investigations are considered later in the chapter.

Retention with overflow

Insidious failure of bladder emptying may lead to chronic retention and, finally, when normal voiding is ineffective, to overflow incontinence. The causes may be:

- lower motor neurone or upper motor neurone lesions;

- urethral obstruction;
- pharmacological.

The patient may be aware of and present with increasing difficulty in bladder emptying or she may present only with frequency. Ultimately, normal emptying stops and a stage of chronic retention with overflow develops.

Symptoms

Symptoms include poor stream, incomplete bladder emptying and straining to void, together with overflow stress incontinence. Often, there will be recurrent urinary tract infection.

Cystometry is usually required to make the diagnosis, and bladder ultrasonography or intravenous or CT (computed tomography) urogram may be necessary to investigate the state of the upper urinary tract to exclude reflux.

Congenital

Epispadias, which is due to faulty midline fusion of mesoderm, results in a widened bladder neck, shortened urethra, separation of the symphysis pubis and imperfect sphincteric control.

The patient complains of stress incontinence which may not be apparent when lying down, but is noticeable when standing up. The physical appearance of epispadias is pathognomonic, and a plain x-ray of the pelvis will show symphysial separation.

It is unlikely that a conventional suprapubic operation to elevate the bladder neck will be sufficient. It may be wiser to proceed straight to urethral reconstruction or an artificial urinary sphincter.

Miscellaneous

Acute urinary tract infection or faecal impaction in the elderly may lead to temporary urinary incontinence. A urethral diverticulum may lead to post-micturition dribble, as urine collects within the diverticulum and escapes as the patient stands up.

Extraurethral causes of incontinence

Congenital

Bladder exstrophy and ectopic ureter

In bladder exstrophy, there is failure of mesodermal migration with breakdown of ectoderm and endoderm, resulting in absence of the anterior abdominal wall and anterior bladder wall. Extensive reconstructive surgery is necessary in the neonatal period.

An ectopic ureter may be single or bilateral and presents with incontinence only if the ectopic opening is outside the bladder, when it may open within the vagina or onto the perineum. The cure is excision of the ectopic ureter and the upper pole of the kidney that it drains.

Fistula

A urinary fistula is an abnormal opening between the urinary tract and the outside (Figure 16.2). Urinary fistulae have obstetric and gynaecological causes. The former include obstructive labour with compression of the bladder between the presenting head and the bony wall of the pelvis. The gynaecological causes are associated with pelvic surgery or pelvic malignancy or radiotherapy.

Whatever the cause, the fistula must be accurately localized. It can be treated by primary closure or by surgery and can be delayed until tissue inflammation and oedema have resolved at about 4 weeks. The surgical techniques involve isolation and removal of the fistula tract, careful debridement, suture and closure of each layer separately and without tension and, if necessary, the interposition of omentum, which brings with it an additional blood supply.

Frequency and urgency

Frequency and urgency are two common urinary symptoms that present singularly or combined. Approximately 15–20 per cent of women have frequency and urgency. Clinical examination and investigation can be directed towards discriminating between the common causes. These include masses that cause compression and prolapse. Investigations should rule out infection, stones and malignancy. A simple urinary diary may show signs of increased fluid intake or evidence of ingestion of too much caffeine and help to diagnose possible diabetes insipidus or mellitus.

Voiding difficulties

Voiding difficulty and acute and chronic urinary retention represent a gradation of failure of bladder emptying. Of women attending a urodynamic clinic, 10–15 per cent may have voiding difficulties. The underlying mechanism is either failure of detrusor contraction or sphincteric relaxation, or urethral obstruction, and this may be due to causes such as stricture and impacted retroverted gravid uterus. Voiding difficulty can also occur after bladder overdistension, such as after pelvic surgery or traumatic vaginal delivery, and careful measurement of any masses that cause compression of the bladder must be excluded and prolapse must be examined for, as this may cause some of the symptoms. If there is vaginal atrophy, this may also cause some urgency and frequency. Volumes voided and post-void residual is recommended to avoid long-term problems.

Symptoms

The main symptoms are poor stream, incomplete emptying and straining to void. As the residual of urine increases in amount, frequency occurs and urinary tract infection develops. Incontinence may follow, and chronic retention and overflow may develop.

Examination

A full bladder may be palpated and there may be the primary signs of the cause of voiding difficulty. Investigations include uroflowmetry, cystometry and

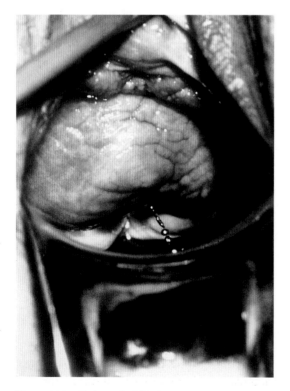

Figure 16.2   Vesicovaginal fistula.

a lumbar sacral spine magnetic resonance imaging (MRI). Part of the assessment involves taking an accurate drug history, as drugs such as anticholinergic agents may have been taken and the patient may be predisposed to retention.

Urinary tract infection

Acute and chronic urinary infections are important and avoidable sources of ill health among women. The short urethra, which is prone to entry of bacteria during intercourse, poor perineal hygiene and the occasional inefficient voiding ability of the patient and unnecessary catheterizations are all contributory factors. Post-menopausal atrophy and change in vaginal pH may predispose to recurrent urinary tract infection (UTI) due to vaginal colonization of coliform bacteria.

A significant urinary infection is defined as the presence of a bacterial count of the same organism/mL of freshly plated urine. On microscopy, there are usually red blood cells and white blood cells. The common organisms are *Escherichia coli, Proteus mirabilis, Klebsiella aerogenes, Pseudomonas aeruginosa* and *Streptococcus faecalis*. These gain entry to the urinary tract by a direct extension from the gut, lymphatic spread via the bloodstream or transurethrally from the perineum. Symptoms include dysuria, frequency and occasionally haematuria. Loin pain and rigors and a temperature above 38°C usually indicate that acute pyelonephritis has developed.

A culture and sensitivity of midstream specimen of urine is required. Intravenous or CT urography or renal ultrasonography may be required in patients with recurrent infection to define anatomical or functional abnormalities.

With acute urinary infection, once a midstream urine specimen has been sent for culture and sensitivity, antimicrobial therapy can begin. If the patient is ill, the treatment should not be delayed and an antimicrobial drug regimen can be started immediately. The regimen can be changed later according to the results of the urine culture and sensitivity. Commonly used drugs include trimethoprim 200 mg twice daily or nitrofurantoin 100 mg four times daily or a cephalosporin.

Recurrent urinary tract infection for which an identifiable source has not been found may be managed by long-term low-dose antimicrobial therapy, such as trimethoprim. Recently, ciprofloxacin and norfloxacin have proved effective. There is sound evidence that vaginal oestrogen treatment can reduce recurrent urinary infections in post-menopausal women.

It is important to treat urinary tract infections effectively, especially in younger women. The development of acute pyelonephritis during pregnancy can be a cause of fetal morbidity.

Investigations

An accurate and detailed history and examination provide a framework for the diagnosis, but there is often a discrepancy between the patient's symptoms and the urodynamic findings. The aim of urodynamic investigations is to provide accurate diagnosis of disorders of micturition and they involve investigation of the lower urinary tract and pelvic floor function.

Investigations range from simple procedures performed in the GP's surgery to sophisticated studies only available in tertiary referral centres. The clinician should pursue a streamlined yet meticulous evaluation, tailoring the investigations to the patient's clinical findings.

Midstream urine specimen

Urinary infection can produce a variety of urinary symptoms, including incontinence. A nitrate stick test can suggest infection, but a diagnosis is made from a clean midstream specimen. The presence of a raised level of white blood cells alone suggests an infection and the test should be repeated. Invasive urodynamics can aggravate infection, and test results are invalid when performed in the presence of infection.

Urinary diary

A urinary diary is a simple record of the patient's fluid intake and output (Figure 16.3). Episodes of urgency and leakage and precipitating events are also recorded. There is no recommended period for diary keeping; a suggested practice is 3–5 consecutive days. These diaries are more accurate than patient recall and provide an assessment of functional bladder capacity. In addition to altering fluid intake, urinary diaries can be utilized to monitor conservative treatment, e.g. bladder re-education, electrical stimulation and drug therapy.

Time	Day 1 Input	Day 1 Output		Day 2 Input	Day 2 Output		Day 3 Input	Day 3 Output
0700 hrs	250	150		200	160	W	250	170
0800 hrs		75	W		50			75
0900 hrs	200	140		200	55		150	60
1000 hrs		100			70			
1100 hrs	150			150		W	200	55
1200 hrs		60	W		100			60
1300 hrs	100	55		100	50			
1400 hrs		75						
1500 hrs			W	100				
1600 hrs	100							
1700 hrs								
1800 hrs								

Figure 16.3   Urinary diary (W, wet episode).

Pad test

Pad tests are used to verify and quantify urine loss. The International Continence Society pad test takes 1 hour. The patient wears a pre-weighed sanitary towel, drinks 500 mL of water and rests for 15 minutes. After a series of defined manoeuvres, the pad is reweighed; a urine loss of more than 1 g is considered significant. If indicated, methylene blue solution can be instilled intravesically prior to the pad test to differentiate between urine and other loss, e.g. insensible loss or vaginal discharge. The popularity of 24-hour and 48-hour pad tests is increasing because they are believed to be more representative. The woman performs normal daily activities and the pad is reweighed after the preferred period.

Uroflowmetry

Uroflowmetry is the measurement of urine flow rate and is a simple, non-invasive procedure that can be performed in the outpatient department (Figure 16.4). It provides an objective measurement of voiding function and the patient can void in privacy.

Although uroflowmetry is performed as part of a general urodynamic assessment, the main indications are complaints of hesitancy or difficulty voiding in patients with neuropathy or a past history of urinary retention. It is also indicated prior to bladder neck or radical pelvic cancer surgery to exclude voiding problems that may deteriorate afterwards.

The normal flow curve is bell shaped. A flow rate <15 mL/second on more than one occasion is

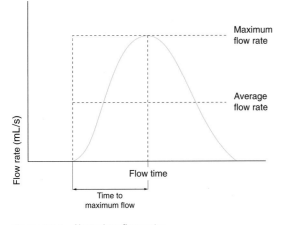

Figure 16.4   Normal uroflowmetry.

considered abnormal in females. The voided volume should be >150 mL, as flow rates with smaller volumes are not reliable. A low peak flow rate and a prolonged voiding time suggest a voiding disorder. Straining can give abnormal flow patterns with interrupted flow. Uroflowmetry alone cannot diagnose the cause of impaired voiding; simultaneous measurement of voiding pressure allows a more detailed assessment.

Cystometry

Cystometry involves the measurement of the pressure–volume relationship of the bladder. It is still considered the most fundamental investigation. It involves simultaneous abdominal pressure recording in addition to intravesical pressure monitoring during bladder filling and voiding. Electronic subtraction of abdominal from intravesical pressure enables determination of the detrusor pressure (Figure 16.5).

Cystometry is indicated for the following:

- Previous unsuccessful continence surgery.
- Multiple symptoms, i.e. urge incontinence, stress incontinence and frequency.
- Voiding disorder.
- Neurogenic bladder.
- Prior to primary continence surgery: this is still debatable if stress incontinence is the only symptom.

Prior to cystometry, the patient voids on the flowmeter. A 12 French gauge catheter is inserted to fill the bladder and any residual urine is recorded. Intravesical pressure is measured using a 1-mm diameter fluid-filled catheter, inserted with the filling line, connected to an external pressure transducer. A fluid-filled 2-mm diameter catheter covered with a rubber finger cot to prevent faecal blockage is inserted into the rectum to measure intra-abdominal pressure. Microtip transducers can be used, but are more expensive and fragile. The bladder is filled (in sitting and standing positions) with a continuous infusion of normal saline at room temperature. The standard filling rate is between 10 and 100 mL/min and is provocative for detrusor instability. During filling, the patient is asked to indicate her first and maximal desire to void and these volumes are noted. The presence of symptoms of urgency and pain and systolic detrusor contractions are noted. Any precipitating factors, such as coughing or running water, are recorded. Pressure rises during filling or standing are also noted. At maximum capacity, the filling line is removed and the patient stands. She is asked to cough and any leakage is documented. The patient then transfers to the uroflowmeter and voids with pressure lines in place. Once urinary flow is established, she is asked to interrupt the flow if possible.

The following are parameters of normal bladder function:

- Residual urine of <50 mL.
- First desire to void between 150 and 200 mL.
- Capacity between 400 and 600 mL.
- Detrusor pressure rise of <15 cmH$_2$O during filling and standing.
- Absence of systolic detrusor contractions.
- No leakage on coughing.
- A voiding detrusor pressure rise of <70 cmH$_2$O with a peak flow rate of >15 mL/second for a volume >150 mL.

Detrusor overactivity is diagnosed when spontaneous or provoked detrusor contractions occur which the patient cannot suppress. Systolic detrusor overactivity is shown by phasic contractions, whereas low compliance detrusor instability is diagnosed when the pressure rise during filling is >15 cmH$_2$O and does not settle when filling ceases. Urodynamic stress incontinence is diagnosed if leakage occurs as a result of coughing in the absence of a rise in detrusor pressure.

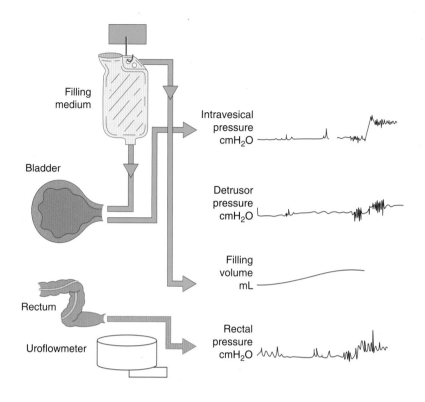

Figure 16.5   Schematic representation of subtracted cystometry.

Videocystourethrography

If a radio-opaque filling medium is used during cystometry, the lower urinary tract can be visualized by x-ray screening with an image intensifier. There are only a few situations in which videocystourethrography (VCU) provides more information than cystometry. During bladder filling, vesicoureteric reflux can be seen. As the screening table is moving to the erect position, any detrusor contraction and leakage can be noted. In the erect position, the patient is asked to cough; bladder neck and base descent and leakage of contrast can be evaluated. During voiding, vesicoureteric reflux, trabeculation and bladder and urethral diverticulae can be noted (Figure 16.6).

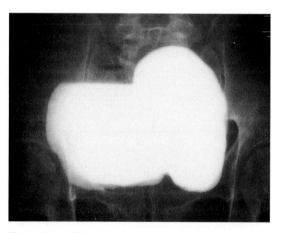

Figure 16.6   Videocystourethrography showing bladder diverticulum.

Intravenous urography

This investigation provides little information about the lower urinary tract, but is indicated in cases of haematuria, neuropathic bladder and suspected ureterovaginal fistula.

Ultrasound

Ultrasound is becoming more widely used in urogynaecology. Post-micturition urine residual estimation can be performed without the need for urethral catheterization and the associated risk of infection. This is useful in the investigation of patients with voiding difficulties, either idiopathic or following postoperative catheter removal. Urethral cysts and diverticula can also be examined using this technique.

Magnetic resonance imaging

Magnetic resonance imaging (MRI) produces accurate anatomical pictures of the pelvic floor and lower urinary tract and has been used to demarcate compartmental prolapse. Although still mostly experimental, the use of endopelvic coils allows fine detail imaging, which may be useful in visualizing damage to the urethral sphincter mechanism.

Cystourethroscopy

Cystourethroscopy establishes the presence of disease in the urethra or bladder. There are few indications in women with incontinence:

- Reduced bladder capacity.
- Short history (less than two years) of urgency and frequency.
- Suspected urethrovaginal or vesicovaginal fistula.
- Haematuria or abnormal cytology.
- Persistent urinary tract infection.

Urethral pressure profilometry

To maintain continence, the urethral pressure must remain higher than the intravesical pressure, and various methods have been devised to measure urethral pressure. Urethral pressure profiles can be obtained using a catheter tip dual sensor microtransducer. Measurement of intraluminal pressure along the urethra at rest or under stress (e.g. coughing) appears to be of little clinical value because of a large overlap between controls and women with USI.

Ambulatory monitoring

During ambulatory monitoring, fine microtip transducers are inserted into the bladder and rectum and data are recorded and stored in a portable device carried by the patient. The pressures are recorded for 4–6 hours with physiological bladder filling and emptying. The data are subsequently downloaded on to computer software and a chart recording is produced. It has become apparent that differences exist between values obtained for artificial and natural filling urodynamic systems in relation to pressure rise during filling and voiding. Ambulatory monitoring appears to be more sensitive than cystometry in the detection of detrusor overactivity.

Treatment

Simple measures, such as exclusion of urinary tract infection, restriction of fluid intake, modifying medication (e.g. diuretics) and treating chronic cough and constipation, play an important role in the management of most types of urinary incontinence.

Urodynamic stress incontinence

Prevention

Shortening the second stage of delivery and reducing traumatic delivery may result in fewer women developing stress incontinence. The benefits of hormone replacement therapy have not been substantiated. The role of pelvic floor exercises either before or during pregnancy needs to be evaluated.

Conservative management

Physiotherapy is the mainstay of the conservative treatment of stress incontinence. The rationale behind pelvic floor education is the reinforcement of cortical awareness of the levator ani muscle group, hypertrophy of existing muscle fibres and a general increase in muscle tone and strength.

With appropriate instruction and regular use, between 40 and 60 per cent of women can derive benefit from pelvic floor exercises to the point where they decline any further intervention.

Pre-menopausal women appear to respond better than their post-menopausal counterparts. Motivation and good compliance are the key factors associated with success. The use of biofeedback techniques, e.g. perineometry and weighted cones, can improve success rates. Maximal electrical stimulation is gaining popularity. A variety of devices have been used but have not been very successful.

Surgery

For women seeking cure, the mainstay of treatment is surgery. The aims of surgery are:

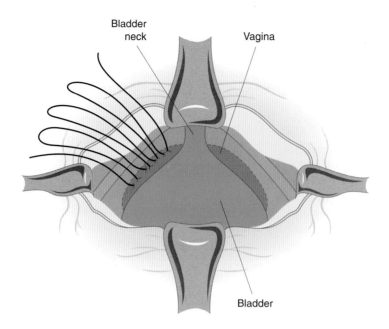

Bladder neck

Vagina

Bladder

Figure 16.7   Diagram showing colposuspension.

- to provide suburethral support;
- restoration of the proximal urethra and bladder neck to the zone of intra-abdominal pressure transmission;
- to increase urethral resistance;
- a combination of both.

The choice of operation depends on the clinical and urodynamic features of each patient, and the route of approach. The colposuspension operation (Figure 16.7) used to be considered the gold standard operation for stress incontinence associated with the highest success rates in the hands of most surgeons. The success rate is over 95 per cent at one year, falling to 78 per cent at 15-year follow up. However, since the introduction of the tension-free vaginal tape (TVT) (Figure 16.8) and subsequent modifications the popularity of the colposuspension has waned.

The original TVT procedure involved the placement of a polypropylene tape under the midurethra through a single 1–2-cm anterior vaginal incision wall incision and two suprapubic 0.5-cm incisions approximately 4–5 cm apart. A needle introducer is passed either side of the urethra through

the vaginal incision and passed through the retropubic space to emerge through the ipsilateral suprapubic incision (Figure 16.9). A cystoscopy is performed to ensure that there is no bladder injury before pulling the needles out through the suprapubic incisions. The tape is attached to both needles and covered in a polythene sheath that allows adjustment. Once adjusted 'tension free', the needles and polythene sheath are removed and the tape trimmed at the

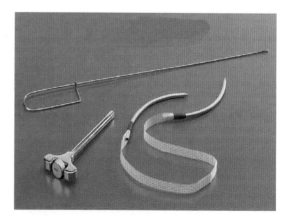

Figure 16.8   Tension-free vaginal tape.

level of the skin. The incisions are then closed with sutures. This procedure has a low complication rate and approximately 90 per cent success rate at one year falling to 80 per cent at ten years. The average return to normal activity is 2 weeks. The midurethral tape procedures have become the most popular surgical treatment for stress incontinence.

Subsequent modifications of the TVT have involved a departure from the retropubic approach to the external incisions being made lateral to the labia over the obturator foramina bilaterally, with early evidence suggesting this approach is equally effective as the retropubic one (Figure 16.10). There is a higher incidence of chronic pain but further evaluation is ongoing.

For the elderly or frail patient with a scarred, narrowed vagina, a bladder neck bulking injection may be more appropriate because it is less invasive and is performed as an office or day-case procedure. Laparoscopic colposuspension may be performed, and in the best hands gives equivalent results to the open procedure but takes longer and does not appear to offer advantages in terms of postoperative recovery.

When the bladder neck is adequately elevated and aligned with the symphysis pubis, it is presumed that the incontinence is due to a defect in the sphincteric mechanism producing a low-resistance, poorly functioning, drainpipe urethra. The procedures to increase outflow resistance in these circumstances are the artificial urinary sphincter and periurethral injections, but suburethral slings are also used.

The artificial sphincter has been used since 1972. It is used where conventional surgery has failed and the patient is mentally alert and manually dexterous. It is a major procedure, performed only in tertiary referral centres because of the level of expertise required. Most of the procedures have been performed on patients with neuropathic bladders, but success rates for persistent female stress incontinence range from 66 to 85 per cent.

Periurethral bulking has attracted considerable interest because of the inherent simplicity of the technique, its applicability in cases where other surgery has failed and its use in the frail patient. With increasing consumer demand, it is being used as a first-line surgical therapy for stress incontinence. Contigen collagen, subcutaneous fat and microparticulate silicon (Macroplastique) have all been evaluated in the last decade. Subcutaneous fat, although cheap, has poor efficacy and therefore has lost popularity.

Contigen collagen is usually injected para-urethrally and Macroplastique transurethrally. Most surgeons inject collagen under local anaesthetic and Macroplastique under general anaesthetic. The principle is to inject the agents into the periurethral tissues at the level of the bladder neck, aiming for bladder neck coaptation (Figure 16.11).

Early success at three-month follow up ranges from 80 to 90 per cent, but there is a time-dependent decline to approximately 50 per cent at three to four years. Complications are uncommon and minor. Dysuria, urinary tract infection and retention requiring overnight catheterization are occasionally encountered. Newer bulking agents are also being utilized. When injectables fail, other bladder neck surgery can be performed without additional problems.

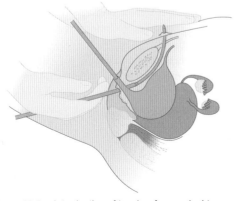

Figure 16.9   Introduction of tension-free vaginal tape trocar.

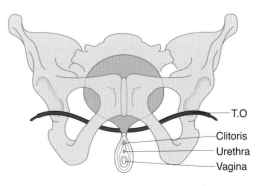

T.O
Clitoris
Urethra
Vagina

Figure 16.10   Transobturator tape.

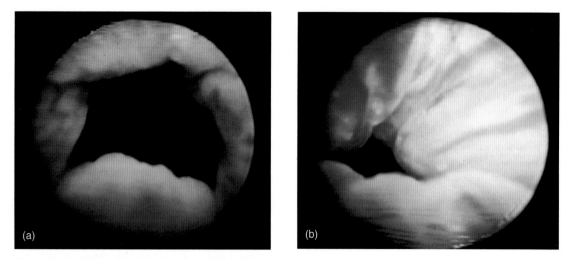

Figure 16.11   The bladder neck (a) before and (b) after collagen injection.

The move towards evidence-based medicine has shown TVT and colposuspension to be the most widely practised and most effective operation for stress incontinence. The anterior repair and endoscopic bladder neck suspensions are not good operations in the medium or long term for this condition. The most important point is that the primary operation provides the best chance of achieving success, as the success rate falls with subsequent attempts.

Detrusor overactivity and voiding difficulty

Detrusor overactivity (DOA) can be treated by bladder retraining, biofeedback or hypnosis, all of which tend to increase the interval between voids and inhibit the symptoms of urgency. These methods are effective in between 60 and 70 per cent of individuals. Anticholinergic agents, such as oxybutynin 2.5 mg twice daily or tolterodine 2 mg twice daily, can be equally as effective. The latter has fewer side effects, mainly dry mouth and constipation. Newer anticholinergic drugs include solifenacin, fesoterodine and darifenacin and these are used regularly as first- and second-line agents for the mangement of DOA. Imipramine is often used for enuresis and desmopressin (an antidiuretic hormone analogue) is useful for nocturia.

Neurogenic and non-neurogenic detrusor instability can be treated with anticholinergic drugs, and when symptoms are resistant, intravesical therapy can be used.

When drug treatments fail, many patients choose to live with pads and appliances but most are not keen on an indwelling urethral or suprapubic catheter. Until recently, the only surgical options were bladder augmentation or ileal conduit.

The introduction of the sacral nerve stimulator offers another alternative. If temporary stimulation of the S3 nerve root with a needle electrode results in symptomatic improvement then a permanent implant can be considered. The technique is expensive and availability limited.

Bladder emptying can be achieved either by the use of clean intermittent self-catheterization or by an indwelling suprapubic or urethral catheter. Drug therapy to encourage and aid detrusor contraction or relax the urethral sphincter is relatively ineffective.

New developments

Single incision tapes are evolving and a few varieties are undergoing evaluation. Figure 16.12 shows one example. These are new suburethral tapes for stress incontinence that do not require external incisions. The tapes are inserted through a vaginal incision and attached to either the obturator internus muscle or into the obturator membrane. If proven to be successful, stress incontinence surgery could be performed under local anaesthetic.

Botulinum toxin injections under cystoscopic control into the detrusor muscle are being used for women with DOA refractory to drug treatment. Early results are encouraging and offer what appears to be an effective alternative to major surgery.

CASE HISTORY

Mrs U is a 54-year-old married Caucasian weighing 95 kg. She is a non-smoker and works as a library administrator.

She presents with a long history of stress incontinence, since the birth of her first child, which has worsened recently. She also has urgency and urge incontinence, but these are not as severe as the stress incontinence. She has daytime frequency and nocturia but no history of voiding difficulty. She has had a previous total abdominal hysterectomy for menorrhagia.

Mrs U has four children; the first was a forceps delivery. The heaviest birthweight was 4 kg.

She is very fit and well but drinks a lot of coffee. She is sexually active.

Examination reveals a normal vaginal capacity and mobility, the bladder neck can be elevated and there is no sign of any major prolapse.

Discussion

What is the most likely diagnosis?

This patient has mixed symptoms but probably has urodynamic stress incontinence. Urodynamics will help to elucidate the cause.

What treatments can she be offered?

Conservative measures would include weight loss and also reduction in caffeine intake. It would be beneficial to advise her about pelvic floor exercises first, before considering surgery. If surgery was to be considered, as the bladder neck can be elevated, the operation of choice might be a colposuspension or TVT. Anterior repair carries much lower success rates and therefore should not be considered.

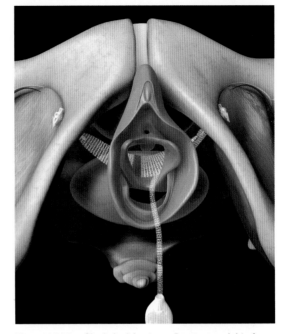

Figure 16.12   Single incision tape. (Image copyright of Bard Inc., 2010.)

Key Points

- Urinary incontinence has a high prevalence, affecting approximately 20–30 per cent of the adult female population.
- The most common causes are USI and detrusor overactivity.
- The mainstays of treatment for USI are physiotherapy and surgery.
- The most appropriate treatment for detrusor overactivity includes bladder retraining and anticholinergic medication.
- Urinary tract infection must always be excluded, as it can cause most urinary symptoms.
- Women with voiding difficulty may present with similar symptoms to women with USI or detrusor overactivity.
- Subtracted cystometry is the most useful investigation for the management of the incontinent patient.
- Surgery for incontinence should be the patient's choice and must be tailored to clinical and urodynamic findings.

Additional reading

Shaw R, Luesley D, Monga A (eds). Urogynaecology section. *Gynaecology*, 4th edn. London: Churchill Livingstone, 2010.

OVERVIEW

Pelvic organ prolapse (POP) is the descent of the genital organs beyond their normal anatomical confines. It is caused by herniation through deficient pelvic fascia or due to weaknesses or deficiency of the ligaments or muscles or blood or nerve supply to the pelvic organs. Most studies are cross-sectional and therefore look at prevalence. The incidence and natural history of the condition is not well understood as there is a lack of prospective longitudinal data. Conservative management involves the use of pessaries, but surgery is the most appropriate option for the physically fit woman.

Definition

A prolapse is a protrusion of an organ or structure beyond its normal confines (Figure 17.1). Prolapses are classified according to their location and the organs contained within them.

Classification

Anterior vaginal wall prolapse

- Urethrocele: urethral descent
- Cystocele: bladder descent
- Cystourethrocele: descent of bladder and urethra

Posterior vaginal wall prolapse

- Rectocele: rectal descent
- Enterocele: small bowel descent

Apical vaginal prolapse

- Uterovaginal: uterine descent with inversion of vaginal apex
- Vault: post-hysterectomy inversion of vaginal apex

Prevalence

Pelvic organ prolapse is a very common problem with a prevalence of 41–50 per cent of women over the age of 40 years. There is a lifetime risk of 7 per cent of having an operation for prolapse and a lifetime risk of 11 per cent of having an operation for incontinence or prolapse. The annual incidence of surgery for POP is within the range of 15–49 cases per 10 000 women years, and it is likely to double in the next 30 years.

Grading

Three degrees of prolapse are described and the lowest or most dependent portion of the prolapse is assessed while the patient is straining:

- 1st: descent within the vagina
- 2nd: descent to the introitus
- 3rd: descent outside the introitus.

In the case of uterovaginal prolapse, the most dependent portion of the prolapse is the cervix, and careful examination can differentiate uterovaginal descent from a long cervix. Third-degree uterine prolapse is termed 'procidentia' and is usually accompanied by cystourethrocele and rectocele.

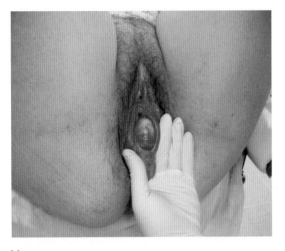

(a)

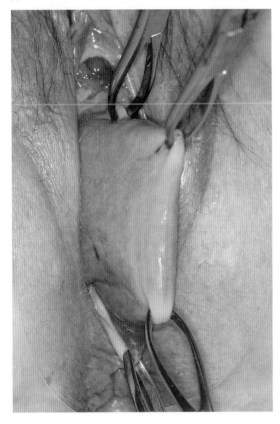

(b)

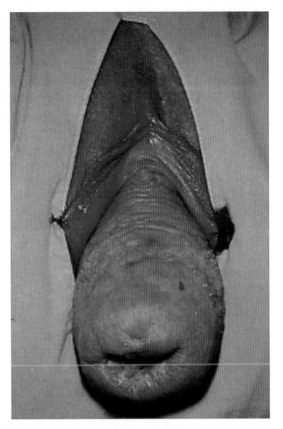

(c)

Figure 17.1   (a) A rectocele; (b) vault prolapse;
(c) uterovaginal prolapse.

Aetiology

The connective tissue, levator ani and intact nerve
supply are vital for the maintenance of position of the
pelvic structures, and are influenced by pregnancy,
childbirth and ageing. Whether congenital or
acquired, connective tissue defects appear to be
important in the aetiology of prolapse and urinary
stress incontinence.

Congenital

Two per cent of symptomatic prolapse occurs in
nulliparous women, implying that there may be a
congenital weakness of connective tissue. In addition,
genital prolapse is rare in Afro-Caribbean women,
suggesting that genetic differences exist.

Childbirth and raised intra-abdominal pressure

The single major factor leading to the development of
genital prolapse appears to be vaginal delivery. Studies

of the levator ani and fascia have shown evidence of nerve and mechanical damage in women with prolapse, compared to those without, occurring as a result of vaginal delivery.

Parity is associated with increasing prolapse. The World Health Organization (WHO) Population Report (1984) suggested that prolapse was up to seven times more common in women who had more than seven children compared to those who had one. Prolapse occurring during pregnancy is rare, but is thought to be mediated by the effects of progesterone and relaxin. In addition, the increase in intra-abdominal pressure will put an added strain on the pelvic floor and a raised intra-abdominal pressure outside pregnancy (e.g. chronic cough or constipation) is also a risk factor.

Ageing

The process of ageing can result in loss of collagen and weakness of fascia and connective tissue. These effects are noted particularly during the post-menopause as a consequence of oestrogen deficiency.

Postoperative

Poor attention to vaginal vault support at the time of hysterectomy leads to vault prolapse in approximately 1 per cent of cases. Mechanical displacement as a result of gynaecological surgery, such as colposuspension, may lead to the development of a rectocele or enterocele.

Clinical features

History

Women usually present with non-specific symptoms. Specific symptoms may help to determine the type of prolapse. Aetiological factors should be enquired about.

Abdominal examination should be performed to exclude organomegaly or abdominopelvic mass.

Symptoms

- **Non-specific**: lump, local discomfort, backache, bleeding/infection if ulcerated, dyspareunia or apareunia. Rarely, in extremely severe cystourethrocele, uterovaginal or vault prolapse, renal failure may occur as a result of ureteric kinking.
- **Specific**:
  - cystourethrocele – urinary frequency and urgency, voiding difficulty, urinary tract infection, stress incontinence;
  - rectocele: incomplete bowel emptying, digitation, splinting, passive anal incontinence.

Vaginal examination

Prolapse may be obvious when examining the patient in the dorsal position if it protrudes beyond the introitus; ulceration and/or atrophy may be apparent.

Understanding the pathophysiology

There are three components that are responsible for supporting the position of the uterus and vagina:

- ligaments and fascia, by suspension from the pelvic side walls;
- levator ani muscles, by constricting and thereby maintaining organ position;
- posterior angulation of the vagina, which is enhanced by rises in abdominal pressure causing closure of the 'flap valve'.

Damage to any of these mechanisms will contribute to prolapse.

Endopelvic fascia is derived from the paramesonephric ducts and is histologically distinct from the fascia investing the pelvic musculature, although attachments exist between the two.

It is a continuous sheet that attaches laterally to the arcus tendineus fascia pelvis and levator ani muscles and extends from the symphysis pubis to the ischial spines. This network of tissue lies immediately beneath the peritoneum, surrounds the viscera and fills the space between the peritoneum above and the levators below; in parts it thickens to form ligaments, e.g. the uterosacral–cardinal complex. This complex is probably the most important component of the support. The segment of fascia that supports the bladder and lies between the bladder and vagina is known as the pubocervical fascia, and that which prevents anterior rectal protrusion and lies between the rectum and posterior vagina is termed the rectovaginal fascia.

(The levator muscles are described in Chapter 1, The gynaecological history and examination.)

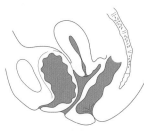
(a) Cystourethrocele

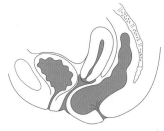
(b) Rectocele

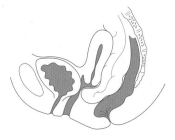
(c) Enterocele

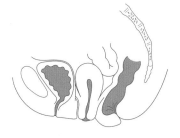
(d) Uterine prolapse

(e) Procidentia

Figure 17.2   Varieties of prolapse.

Vaginal pelvic examination should be performed and pelvic mass excluded.

The anterior and posterior vaginal walls and cervical descent should be assessed with the patient straining in the left lateral position, using a Sims speculum. Combined rectal and vaginal digital examination can be an aid to differentiate rectocele from enterocele (Figure 17.2).

Differential diagnosis

- Anterior wall prolapse: congenital or inclusion dermoid vaginal cyst, urethral diverticulum.
- Uterovaginal prolapse: large uterine polyp.

Treatment

The choice of treatment depends on the patient's wishes, level of fitness and desire to preserve coital function.

Prior to specific treatment, attempts should be made to correct obesity, chronic cough or

Investigations

There are no essential investigations. If urinary symptoms are present, urine microscopy, cystometry and cystoscopy should be considered. The relationship between urinary symptoms and prolapse is complex. Some women with cystourethrocele have concurrent incontinence; as the prolapse increases in severity, urethral kinking may restore continence but lead to voiding difficulty (see Chapter 16, Urogynaecology). Should renal failure be suspected, serum urea and creatinine should be evaluated and renal ultrasound performed. For women with symptoms of obstructed defaecation MR proctography can help diagnose a rectocele (Figure 17.3).

constipation. If the prolapse is ulcerated, a 7-day course of topical oestrogen should be administered.

Prevention

Shortening the second stage of delivery and reducing traumatic delivery may result in fewer women developing a prolapse. The benefits of episiotomy and hormone replacement therapy at the menopause have not been substantiated.

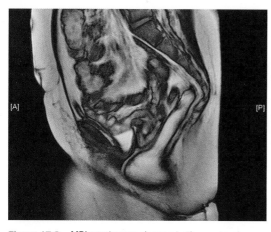

Figure 17.3   MRI proctogram demonstrating rectocele.

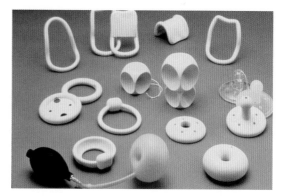

Figure 17.5   New range of pessaries.

Medical

If a woman is found to have uterovaginal prolapse on examination but has no symptoms, then it would be inappropriate to offer any surgical treatment and either observation or conservative therapy would be best. If symptoms are mild, then pelvic floor physiotherapy is offered but there are no randomized controlled trials examining the effectiveness of physiotherapy on prolapse. Silicon rubber-based ring pessaries are the most popular form of conservative therapy. They are inserted into the vagina in much the same way as a contraceptive diaphragm and need replacement at annual intervals (Figure 17.4). Shelf pessaries are rarely used but may be useful in women who cannot retain a ring pessary. The use of pessaries can be complicated by vaginal ulceration and infection. The vagina should therefore be carefully inspected at the time of replacement. There are a whole range of newer pessaries that are undergoing evaluation and these may be more comfortable for the patient (Figure 17.5).

Indications for pessary treatment are:

- patient's wish;
- as a therapeutic test;
- childbearing not complete;
- medically unfit;
- during and after pregnancy (awaiting involution);
- while awaiting surgery.

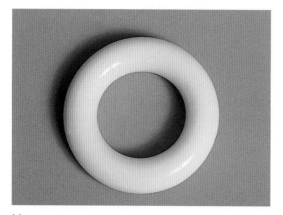

(a)

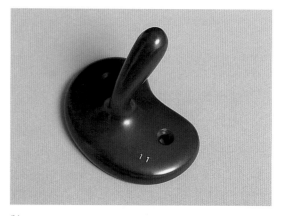

(b)

Figure 17.4   (a) Ring pessary and (b) shelf pessary.

Surgery

The aim of surgical repair is to restore anatomy and function. There are vaginal and abdominal operations designed to correct prolapse, and choice often depends on a woman's desire to preserve coital function (Figure 17.6).

Cystourethrocele

Anterior repair (colporrhaphy) is the most commonly performed surgical procedure but should be avoided if there is concurrent stress incontinence. An anterior vaginal wall incision is made and the fascial defect allowing the bladder to herniate through is identified and closed. With the bladder position restored, any redundant vaginal epithelium is excised and the incision closed.

Rectocele

Posterior repair (colporrhaphy) is the most commonly performed procedure. A posterior vaginal wall incision is made and the fascial defect allowing the rectum to herniate through is identified and closed. With the rectal position restored, any redundant vaginal epithelium is excised and the incision closed.

Enterocele

The surgical principles are similar to those of anterior and posterior repair, but the peritoneal sac containing the small bowel should be excised. In addition, the pouch of Douglas is closed by approximating the peritoneum and/or the uterosacral ligaments.

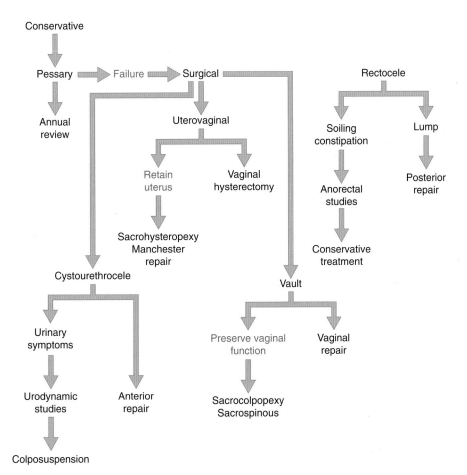

Figure 17.6 Treatment of prolapse.

Uterovaginal prolapse

Uterine preserving surgery

Uterine preserving surgery is used largely when a woman still wants to have further children and therefore the uterus has to be preserved. Occasionally, a woman wishes to preserve her uterus and then may choose this option:

- **Hysterosacropexy:** This may be performed by an open route or a laparoscopic route and a mesh is attached to the isthmus of the cervix and the uterus is suspended by attaching the other part of the mesh to the anterior longitudinal ligament on the sacrum.

- **The Manchester repair:** This involves accessing the uterus vaginally amputating the cervix and using the uterosacral cardinal ligament complex to support the uterus. The operation is rarely used now because of problems with complications to the cervix resulting in either cervical stenosis or cervical incompetence and a risk of miscarriage.

- **Le Fort colpocleisis:** This operation is used in very frail patients who are unfit for major surgery and are not sexually active. It involves partial closure of the vagina while preserving the uterus.

- **'Total mesh' procedure using an introducer device (Figure 17.7):** There is a range of mesh using devices that have been designed not only for anterior and posterior vaginal prolapse but suggest they may be useful in uterovaginal prolapse and can preserve the uterus. The data for this is scarce.

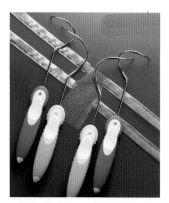

Figure 17.7   New mesh kit for prolapse.

Procedures involving hysterectomy

These procedures involve removal of the uterus:

- **Vaginal hysterectomy:** This is one of the oldest major operations with references dating from the time of Hypocrates in the fifth century BC. The operation involves making an incision around the cervix and entering the peritoneal cavity from the vaginal side ligating all the major blood vessels and delivering the uterus through the vagina and suturing the vault of the vagina. Obviously, there is lack of support of the vault and to try and improve support, the standard procedure is to shorten the stretched uterosacral cardinal ligament complex and then resuture into the vault of the vagina. Some authors have used variations of this to try and attach the vault even higher in the vagina with a higher uterosacral ligament fixation. A number of modifications have been suggested to try and improve the support of the vagina. Some surgeons use laparoscopically assisted techniques to perform a vaginal hysterectomy if there is abdominal pathology, but this is not usual for prolapse.

- **Total abdominal hysterectomy and sacrocolpopexy:** This involves complete removal of the uterus through an abdominal incision, followed by repair of the vault of the vagina and then attaching a mesh to the vault of the vagina and suspending it to the anterior longitudinal ligament on the sacrum. Opening the vagina at the time of inserting a mesh greatly increases the risk of vaginal erosion and therefore this procedure is not commonly practised.

- **Subtotal abdominal hysterectomy and sacrocervicopexy:** This operation is becoming more popular. It involves either an abdominal or laparoscopic approach. Most surgeons use the abdominal route. A subtotal hysterectomy is performed leaving the cervix intact. This means the vagina is not entered and there is no vaginal scarring. The cervix is then used as an attachment point for the mesh where there is negligible chance of erosion and the mesh is suspended to the anterior longitudinal ligament on the sacrum.

If there is concomitant anterior prolapse at the time of vaginal hysterectomy an anterior repair may be performed. If there is concomitant anterior prolapse at the time of an abdominal procedure a paravaginal repair can be performed, again avoiding the need for an incision in the vagina.

Vault prolapse

Sacrocolpopexy (Figure 17.8) is similar to sacrohysteropexy but the inverted vaginal vault is attached to the sacrum using a mesh and the pouch of Douglas is closed. Sacrospinous ligament fixation is a vaginal procedure in which the vault is sutured to one or other sacrospinous ligament.

Key Points

- A prolapse is a protrusion of an organ or structure beyond its normal confines; prolapses are extremely common in multiparous women.
- Damage to the major supports of the vagina, i.e. ligaments, fascia and levator ani muscles, leads to prolapse.
- Childbirth injury is the major aetiological factor.
- Most women with prolapse present with non-specific symptoms, such as a lump and backache.
- Women with cystourethrocele often have urinary symptoms.
- Women with rectocele often have bowel symptoms.
- Diagnosis is made by clinical examination.
- Surgery is the mainstay of treatment.

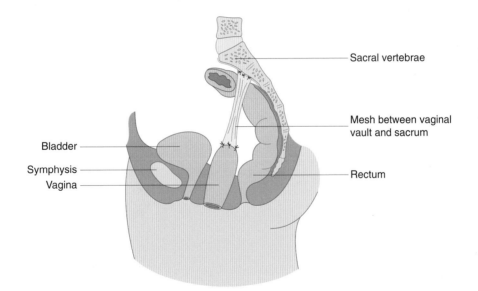

Figure 17.8   Sacrocolpopexy.

CASE HISTORY

Mrs PS is a 48-year-old married, sexually active Caucasian, weighing 89 kg. She is a non-smoker and works as a nursing assistant in a nursing home. She suffers from asthma and uses salbutamol and Becloforte inhalers.

She presents with an eight-month history of 'feeling a lump down below' and backache. The lump is bigger when she has been on her feet all day. She also complains of poor urinary stream and a feeling of incomplete emptying of her bladder. She admits to no urinary incontinence or bowel symptoms. She had a total abdominal hysterectomy three years previously for menorrhagia.

Mrs PS has two children, aged 22 and 24 years. Both were delivered vaginally; the heaviest at birth weighed 3.8 kg.

Discussion

What is the most likely diagnosis?

Anterior vaginal wall prolapse is the most likely diagnosis in view of her urinary symptoms. However, vault prolapse and rectocele can also cause obstructive urinary symptoms.

What risk factors does she have for the development of prolapse?

- Vaginal delivery of a large infant can cause damage to pelvic nerves, endopelvic fascia and levator ani, which can result in prolapse.

- She is overweight and this will increase the effect of abdominal pressure on the pelvic floor.

- She has a chronic cough and her job involves heavy lifting. Both these factors increase abdominal pressure.

Additional reading

Shaw R, Luesley D, Monga A (eds). Urogynaecology section. *Gynaecology*, 4th edn. London: Churchill Livingstone, 2010.

THE MENOPAUSE

OVERVIEW

The average age of the menopause in Western women is approximately 52 years, a figure which has remained remarkably consistent over the last few hundred years (Figure 18.1). However, during this time the average life expectancy has increased steadily with many women now living well into their 80s and beyond. Women can now expect to live over a third of their life after the menopause, and consequently over the last 40 years or so there has been an increasing interest in the effects of the menopause on long-term health, its effects on quality of life and the potential treatments.

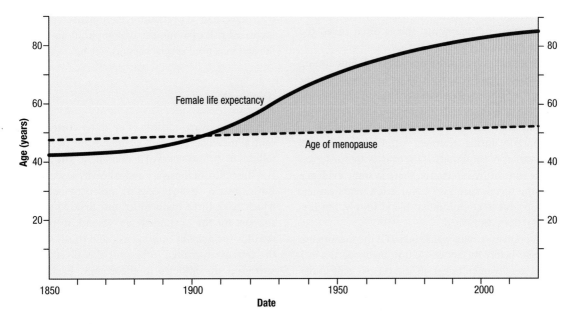

Figure 18.1　Age of menopause and age of mean life expectancy in the UK since 1850.

Definitions

The term 'menopause' means the final menstrual period (from the Greek *menos* (month) and *pausos* (ending)) and represents a watershed in the reproductive life of a woman. The term 'menopause' was first coined in early nineteenth century France at a time of radical social reform. In Victorian Britain, there was little interest until around 1860.

The term 'climacteric' (from the Greek *klimakter* (rung of a ladder)) signifies a major movement on life's ladder and is often used synonymously with 'perimenopause' or 'the change'. It marks the transition from the reproductive to the non-reproductive state, the menopause being a specific event within that phase.

The menopause occurs as a result of loss of ovarian follicular activity leading to a fall in oestradiol levels below the level needed for endometrial stimulation. Strictly speaking, it can only be said to have occurred after 12 consecutive months of amenorrhoea. While the menopause can sometimes be a sudden event, for most women there is a gradual change in menstrual pattern in the years preceding the menopause as ovarian activity fluctuates, which may be accompanied by troublesome symptoms; this is often called the 'perimenopause'.

A surgical menopause occurs when functioning ovaries are removed, such as at hysterectomy for malignancy or severe endometriosis. A menopause may also be iatrogenically induced by other treatments, such as radio- or chemotherapy, for malignancy or temporarily during treatment with GnRH analogues for a variety of conditions. If the ovaries are conserved at the time of hysterectomy, there is some evidence that the menopause may occur a few years earlier, perhaps due to compromised blood supply, but this has not been confirmed.

A premature menopause occurs if the menopause happens before the age of 45. It probably occurs in 1 per cent of women under 40 and 0.1 per cent under 30. It is one of the more common causes of primary and secondary amenorrhoea and should always be considered in the diagnosis. The cause of spontaneous premature ovarian failure is usually unknown, but there are a number of well-established causes that should be excluded (Table 18.1). Either there may be something wrong with the ovaries themselves (primary ovarian failure), e.g. certain chromosomal abnormalities or autoimmune disorders, or something

Table 18.1   Principle causes of premature ovarian failure

Primary	Chromosome anomalies, e.g. Turner's, Fragile X
	Auto-immune disease, e.g. hypothyroidism, Addison's, myasthenia gravis
	Enzyme deficiencies, e.g. galactosaemia, 17α-hydroxylase deficiency
Secondary	Surgical menopause after bilateral oophorectomy
	Chemotherapy or radiotherapy
	Infections, e.g. tuberculosis, mumps, malaria, varicella

happens to the ovary, e.g. oophorectomy or damage following radio- or chemotherapy. With an increasing number of women surviving childhood cancers, this latter group are becoming more prevalent. Women who have had a premature menopause are at an increased risk of a number of complications later in life and may need special support (see below).

Pathophysiology

The human ovary consists of an outer cortex and a central medulla. The cortex contains the developing follicles in various stages of development. The medulla is at the centre of the ovary and is heavily vascularized. Both contain stromal cells of mesenchymal origin which have three main functions: first, to provide support for the ovarian tissue; second, to produce steroids (principally androgens), and third, some of the cells are recruited to become thecal cells which surround the follicles in the cortex. Each ovary contains several million germ cell units (primordial follicles or oocytes) which achieve maximal levels of about 1.5 million *in utero*. There is a steady decline in these units over the prepubertal and reproductive years (Figure 18.2), but the maturation of some of these follicular units during this time is one of the key components of ovulation, corpus luteum formation and ovarian steroidogenesis. It is estimated that for every follicle which matures to ovulation, up to 1000

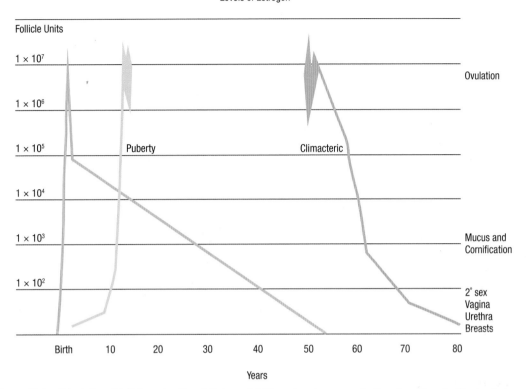

Figure 18.2   Correlation of follicle maturation, follicle availability and oestrogen production. Reproduced with permission from Speroff L, Glass RH, Kase NG. *Clinical gynecologic endocrinology and infertility.* Baltimore, MD: Williams & Wilkins, 1990: 121–64.

follicles fail and become atretic and probably only 400 of the 400 000 follicles present at puberty ever mature to ovulation.

The ovaries produce four principal steroid hormones: oestradiol, progesterone and the androgens, testosterone and androstenedione. Ovarian function and the normal menstrual cycle are controlled by the gonadotrophins follicle-stimulating hormone (FSH) and luteinizing hormone (LH), which are released from the anterior pituitary gland. Their release is controlled by the release of gonadotrophin-releasing hormone (GnRH) from the hypothalamus, which in turn is governed by the negative feedback from circulating levels of oestradiol, progesterone and inhibin (a peptide hormone produced by the ovary). The majority of circulating plasma oestradiol in premenopausal women is produced from the developing follicle. Oestradiol synthesis is principally

from conversion of androstenedione and testosterone, which occurs in the granulosa cells that line the developing follicle. The conversion is catalysed by the aromatase enzyme cascade and is stimulated by FSH. Oestradiol is also converted in the theca cells from androgens, which in turn are created from cholesterol under the direct stimulation of LH. Mean plasma levels fluctuate widely throughout the cycle (Figure 18.2) with a median level of 4–500 pmol/L.

As the ovary ages the remaining follicles, which are probably the least sensitive to gonadotrophins, are increasingly less likely to mature and so ovulation declines and ovarian function gradually fails. The first endocrine change is a fall in inhibin production by the ovary. Inhibin is a glycoprotein that inhibits production of FSH from the anterior pituitary, hence with loss of this control plasma FSH levels start to rise. Eventually, the level of oestradiol production

Investigations

The cessation of cyclical menstrual bleeding varies. A woman may experience a gradual change in her menstrual cycle over several months or even years in her late 40s or early 50s before the bleeding ceases altogether. This may be accompanied by classical menopausal symptoms. Other women may have an abrupt cessation of their cycles without any warning, while some women have episodes of oligomenorrhoea with an occasional cycle. In these situations, the diagnosis is pretty straightforward and does not require specific investigation. However, in other clinical situations, it can be helpful to confirm the diagnosis or perhaps more commonly to refute the diagnosis, for example in a woman in her mid 40s with vague symptoms who thinks she is going through the menopause. Here, a normal FSH/LH levels will help to reassure that this is not the cause. It is mandatory, however, to investigate women suspected of undergoing a premature menopause. The implications of the diagnosis have major long-term consequences, both in terms of long-term treatment and also potential fertility. The younger women (under 40 years) require detailed assessment and specialist assessment.

What investigations

FSH measurements are the most useful for confirming the diagnosis. A level of >30 IU/L is considered diagnostic of menopause. However, there is significant daily variation of FSH levels throughout the cycle and the results should be interpreted with caution and repeated if necessary. The tests are best done on day 3–5 of the cycle when FSH levels are usually at their lowest. To confirm that a woman with amenorrhoea or who has been hysterectomized is menopausal, two measurements at least 2 weeks and up to three months apart are recommended. FSH levels are of no use at predicting when menopause will occur or assessing fertility status. Equally, monitoring FSH levels on treatment is of little value. There is no value in using oestradiol, progesterone, testosterone or LH levels in the diagnosis of menopause. Oestradiol levels may be useful in monitoring treatment in certain situations.

Thyroid function (T4 and TSH) should be checked if there are any clinical suspicions as the symptoms of hypothyroidism can be confused with menopause or may explain poor response to oestrogens. In resistant cases of intractable hot flushes, 24-hour urinary collections of catecholamines (VMA), 5-hydroxyindolactetic acid (5HIAA) and methlyhistamine may be done to exclude rare causes, such as phaeochromocytoma, carcinoid syndrome and mastocytosis, respectively.

Further assessment

The menopause presents an opportunity to screen for significant disease in later years and introduce appropriate preventative measures. There a wide range of investigations that can be performed:

- Breast screening and mammography
- Endometrial assessment of unschedulded bleeding
- Cardiovascular disease risk assessment
- Skeletal assessment including bone density estimation and fracture risk assessment.

is no longer sufficient to stimulate endometrial proliferation and menopause ensues. Further decline in oestradiol levels over subsequent years has effects on all oestrogen-responsive tissues (which are widespread throughout the body, see below). As a result, the effects of ovarian failure are often noted before the last period and the effects can go on for many years. Menopause may only be a single event, but it represents a significant change in a woman's hormonal milieu which has implications for her future health and quality of life – hence the importance of post-reproductive health for women.

Effects of the menopause

The menopause has a significant impact throughout the body but individual women's experiences will vary enormously. Some women have no symptoms at all, while others can have a dreadful time with debilitating symptoms that stop them functioning properly. The effects vary chronologically and are summarized in Table 18.2.

Genitourinary problems

Urogenital atrophy is a common observation in postmenopausal women which increases with age, but the prevalence of symptomatic atrophy is unclear. In a population-based study of Australian women observed over seven years, vaginal dryness was a complaint in 3 per cent of premenopausal women, 4 per cent of women in early menopause, but up to 47 per cent of women three years or more into their menopause. Vaginal atrophy results in loss of the normal architecture within the vaginal epithelium

Table 18.2   Effects of the menopause in different time frames

Short term (0–5 years)	Vasomotor symptoms, e.g. hot flushes, night sweats
	Psychological symptoms, e.g. labile mood, anxiety, tearfulness
	Loss of concentration, poor memory
	Joint aches and pains
	Dry and itchy skin
	Hair changes
	Decreased sexual desire
Intermediate (3–10 years)	Vaginal dryness, soreness
	Dyspareunia
	Sensory urgency
	Recurrent urinary tract infections
	Urogenital prolapse
Long term (>10 years)	Osteoporosis
	Cardiovascular disease
	Dementia

Menopausal symptoms

Vasomotor symptoms, which usually manifest as hot flushes or night sweats, are the most common symptoms of the menopause. About 70 per cent of women in the West experience some form of vasomotor symptoms, but their intensity varies. Their exact cause is unknown, but it is thought that a relative fall in circulating oestrogen levels disrupts the control of the body's thermostat, located in the hypothalamus, leading to cutaneous vasodilatation and heat loss. Classically, the hot flush only affects the upper trunk and head and neck. Recent renewed interest in the cause of the hot flush has implicated a possible role for serotonin and its receptors in the central nervous system. Certain triggers can be identified, such as stress, spicy foods, alcohol, caffeine and hot drinks, although these are often very individual. Typically, hot flushes start to occur a year or two before the menopause, peaking in frequency and intensity in the first year after menopause and on average lasting for up to five years. However, they can continue for 20 or more years and some unfortunate individuals continue to flush all their lives.

Flushes occurring at night lead to night sweats, which in turn disrupts sleep, which in turn leads to tiredness and can affect mood, concentration and libido.

Symptoms such as irritability, depressed mood, anxiety, loss of memory and concentration, overwhelming tiredness and mood swings are common around the menopause. There is a peak in the number of women who report this type of problem around the menopause, although whether these problems are actually caused by ovarian failure or secondary to other menopausal symptoms, or due to other co-existing factors is questionable. Women who report psychological symptoms at the menopause are more likely to have had previous psychological problems, poor health, other life stresses and a negative attitude to ageing. In Western society, the woman is often the lynchpin that keeps many families together and the menopause usually occurs at a time of life when there can be many other stressful events going on. The additional physical and emotional changes that occur at the menopause can put this balance under pressure and some women will struggle to cope. Whatever the underlying cause, many women do need additional support during this time and some may benefit from specific treatment for their symptoms, such as hormone replacement therapy (HRT).

(Figure 18.3), reducing its secretions and elasticity and making it more prone to trauma, dryness, spontaneous bleeding and infection. Clinically, this manifests as vaginal dryness, itching, dyspareunia, vaginal pain, discharge, bleeding or vaginal infection.

The distal urethra and trigone of the bladder have a similar embryological origin as the lower vagina and are also prone to atrophy with oestrogen deficiency. This can lead to troublesome urinary symptoms, such as urinary frequency and dysuria, in the absence of proven infection. Sometimes referred to as the 'urethral syndrome', this responds well to vaginal oestrogens. Thinning of the urethral mucosa and trigone results in a more sensitive and trauma-prone bladder which in turn leads to sensory urgency and recurrent urinary tract infections, symptoms that also respond well to local oestrogen administration. Loss of oestrogen also plays a role in

more widespread pelvic floor dysfunction leading to weakening of the supporting tissues and ligaments, which may already be damaged by childbirth or other trauma, and thus contributing to the increased

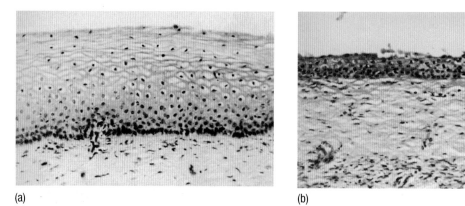

(a)   (b)

Figure 18.3   Vaginal epithelium in (a) premenopausal woman and (b) postmenopausal woman showing atrophic changes. Note the loss of epithelial structure and architecture. Reproduced with permission from *Atlas of the menopause*.

incidence of prolapse and stress urinary incontinence seen after menopause.

Many women complain of loss of sexual desire or libido around the menopause. Whether this is directly due to a fall in oestrogen or other simultaneous factors is now the subject of considerable research. The term 'female sexual dysfunction' is now in widespread use based on a classification system introduced by the International Consensus Development Conference on Female Sexual Dysfunction. One survey highlighted that among 18–59 year olds sexual dysfunction was more prevalent in women (43 per cent) than men (31 per cent) and that the prevalence of sexual dysfunction rose from 42 to 88 per cent during the menopausal transition.

Long-term effects

Oestrogen receptors are widespread throughout the body and the fall in circulating oestradiol levels leads to a number of changes in a variety of organs and systems that can have notable effects on quality of life and a potentially major impact on long-term morbidity and mortality. These conditions often develop without obvious clinical manifestation in the early post-menopause, but pose a significant economic burden for the future particularly with an increasingly ageing population. For women who undergo a premature menopause, the prolonged time they spend without oestrogen increases the risk of these conditions developing at a younger age.

Osteoporosis

Eighty per cent of our skeleton is comprised of cortical bone, the other 20 per cent being trabecular bone. The latter is principally found in the vertebrae, long bones, such as femur and humerus, and the wrist. Trabecular bone has a shock absorbing capacity which is accomplished using its large surface area of interconnecting trabeculae (Figure 18.4). It is constantly undergoing turnover (Figure 18.5) and is oestrogen sensitive. Oestrogen acts as an antiresorptive agent on trabecular bone and the fall in oestrogen levels after the menopause is characterized by an unprecedented fall in bone density (Figure 18.6), which ultimately may lead to an increased risk of osteoporotic fracture. Osteoporosis is defined as 'a skeletal disorder characterized by compromised bone strength predisposing to an increased risk of fracture'. Bone strength is principally a reflection of bone quality and bone density. The latter is clinically more relevant as it can be readily measured and a woman's osteoporotic risk assessed using standard WHO criteria. Osteoporosis is a major health problem for the Western world that will only worsen as the population ages. It is far more prevalent in women than men and it is estimated that as many as 50 per cent of women will suffer an osteoporotic fracture during their lifetime.

Current treatment strategies target preventative treatment at individuals identified as being at high risk of subsequent fracture rather than treating large sections of the population. The FRAX model screens

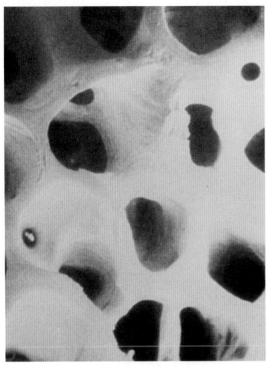

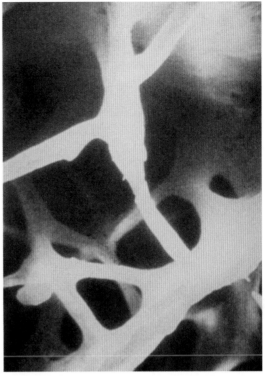

(a)   (b)

Figure 18.4   Electron micrograph of trabecular bone showing (a) normal structure and (b) osteoporotic bone. Note the loss of architecture and density in (b) making the bone weaker and more prone to fracture. Reproduced with permission from *Atlas of the menopause.*

postmenopausal women for risk factors including age at menopause (premature menopause being particularly high risk). Those deemed as increased risk undergo DEXA bone scanning and those with low bone density offered preventative treatment. There is much debate about when to start preventative treatment as long-term treatments have potential adverse effects and are costly. Recent NICE guidance favours a very limited role for preventative treatment in women under 75 years, except those with previous fracture. Prevention of osteoporosis remains a life-long strategy, even if for some or most of that time no specific treatment is used.

Other long-term consequences

While coronary heart disease (CHD) is the single most common cause of death in women in the United Kingdom, it is relatively uncommon before the menopause. There is a large body of evidence suggesting that oestrogen has a protective influence against CHD. Early menopause without additional oestrogen is associated with a two- to four-fold increased risk in CHD and many studies have suggested that taking oestrogens around the time of the menopause reduces CHD risk. Menopause is associated with a number of potentially adverse metabolic changes, such as a rise in total and LDL cholesterol and a fall in HDL cholesterol. These changes are reversed with oestrogen. Oestrogen also has a direct effect on the vessel wall: loss of oestrogen is associated with vasoconstriction and atherogenesis, while oestrogen administration stimulates vasodilatation via nitric oxide.

Dementia is much more common in women, but the evidence for a role of oestrogen and menopause in the pathophysiology of cognitive decline and dementia is conflicting. Many women report memory changes during the menopause and an early menopause is associated with an increased dementia risk in later

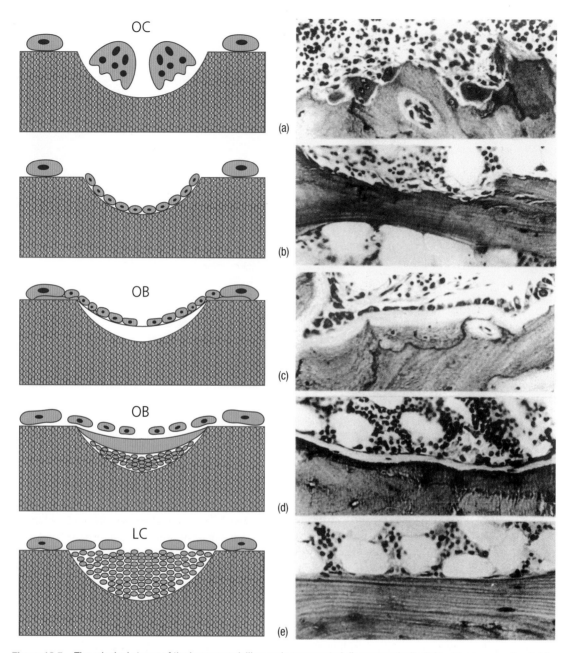

Figure 18.5 The principal stages of the bone remodelling cycle represented diagrammatically (left) with corresponding light micrographs of iliac crest biopsies (right). (a) Resorption by osteoclasts (OC); (b) reversal with disappearance of osteoclasts; (c) formation with the deposition of osteoid by osteoblasts (OB); (d) mineralization of the osteoid; (e) completion of the cycle with bone lining cells on the surface (LC); Light micrographs reproduced with permission from Dempster DW, *Disorders of bone and mineral metabolism*, New York: Raven Press, 1992.

life. Some studies have suggested that oestrogen use around the time of the menopause may improve cognitive function and reduce the risk of Alzheimer's, but others have not confirmed this.

Management

The menopause is a natural event and for many women there is no need to 'manage' it at all, although

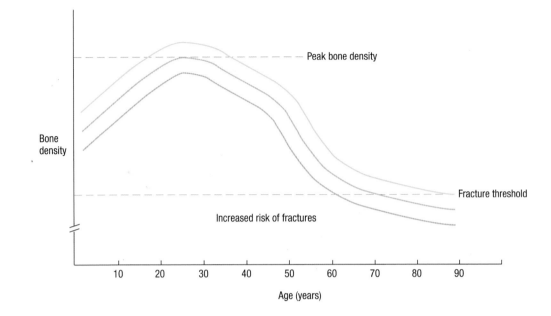

Figure 18.6   Changes in bone density with age and associated fracture risk.

awareness of the long-term implications, such as osteoporosis and cardiovascular disease, should be part of good preventative medicine. However, for other women the menopause can be a difficult time and there are a variety of treatment options available. While HRT is an extremely effective option, it is only one of a number of possible approaches. For most women, menopausal symptoms are relatively short lived and will settle within a few years, but for some they will go on much longer and longer-term treatment may be needed. The menopause is a hormonal milestone and provides an opportunity to establish firm strategies for the prevention of the long-term disorders outlined above. The assessment of the menopausal woman should follow a normal approach with some key aspects.

The menopause consultation

Frequently, enquiries about menopausal symptoms will form part of a more general gynaecological assessment unless in a specialist endocrine or menopause clinic. The history should concentrate on ascertaining the frequency and severity of menopausal symptoms and their impact on day-to-day activities. While many women have symptoms, not all of them are troublesome enough for specific treatment, and all treatments have potential side effects. It must be emphasized that not all women will necessarily link some of their symptoms with the menopause, so direct questioning may be helpful. Equally, enquiry into any sexual problems, in particular vaginal dryness, soreness and bladder symptoms, should be recorded. Any previous treatments and side effects should be noted, including over-the-counter preparations. Family and personal history should focus on risk factors for cardiovascular disease, osteoporosis, breast cancer, thrombosis and ovarian cancer.

Physical examination may well be part of a more generalized gynaecological assessment. In a menopause consultation, it is necessary to exclude co-existent gynaecological problems if these have not already been done. Thus, general breast and abdominal examination, cervical smear and bimanual assessment of uterine size should be performed.

If there are specific urogenital symptoms, then assessment of the vagina for atrophy, prolapse or incontinence is advised.

Lifestyle

For many women, the menopause can be a time of uncertainty and may be the first time they have sought professional help for themselves for many years. It is an ideal time to look at changes in diet and exercise and build for a healthy future to maximize their health potential. Smoking is associated with an earlier menopause, and an increased risk of many serious diseases. Smoking cessation leads to a steady reduction in all the increased risks and should be encouraged as part of a health promotion strategy. It is particularly important for women going through the menopause to eat sensibly and try to avoid excessive weight gain. Body weight increases on average 1 kg per year around menopause. Although this is not a direct effect of the menopause itself, there are changes in body fat distribution that redistributes body fat from the hips and thighs (gynaecoid) to the more android distribution (abdomen). Regular physical activity, even of low intensity, can have positive effects on a variety of conditions. It helps to conserve bone density in the hip and spine, maintain muscle strength, joint flexibility and overall balance, all factors that will reduce the risk of falls and subsequent fracture. It also has a beneficial effect on cardiovascular risk and can be effectively used to reduce vasomotor symptoms.

Alternative and complementary therapies

A wide variety of alternative medicines are used to improve menopausal symptoms (Table 18.3), although there is little evidence for the efficacy and safety of most of them. These products are currently unregulated in the UK and while the majority are likely to be harmless, a number of serious and potentially fatal interactions have been reported between herbal supplements and standard medications. Despite this, the use of such treatments is widespread and increasing. Phyto-oestrogens, which are plant substances with similar activity to oestrogen, do appear to have some beneficial effects on both menopausal symptoms, but their long-term safety is not known.

Table 18.3   List of prescription and non-prescription therapies commonly used in the treatment of menopausal symptoms

Non-prescription	
Lifestyle changes	Diet and exercise
Complementary therapies	Acupuncture
	Reflexology
	Magnetism
Herbal remedies	Black cohosh (Actaea racemosa)
	Dong quai (Angelica sinensis)
	Evening primrose oil (Oenothera biennis)
	Gingko (Gingko biloba)
	Ginseng (Panax ginseng)
	Kava kava (Piper methysticum)
	St John's wort (Hypericum perforatum)
'Bio-identical' hormones	Natural progesterone gel
	DHEA
	Phytoestrogens, e.g. isoflavones, red clover
Prescription	
α-adrenergic agonists	Clonodine
βeta-blockers	Propanolol
Selective serotonin reuptake inhibitors	Venlafaxine, fluoxetine, paroxetine, citalopram
	Gabapentin
Hormone replacement therapy (HRT)	Oestrogen alone
	Oestrogen and progestogen combined
	Progestogen alone

There is limited evidence that some complementary therapies, such as acupuncture or magnetism, may have a role in improving vasomotor symptoms.

Non-hormonal treatments

Some of the selective serotonin-reuptake inhibitors (SSRI) and gabapentin have been shown to improve hot flushes in short trials. However, these products have significant side effects and should only be used for women with intractable symptoms who cannot take HRT (Table 18.3).

For osteoporosis prevention, the bisphosphonates are the principle class of drug used. Alternatives include strontium and Raloxifene®, which is a type of SERM (see below under New developments). However, all these can have significant side effects and should usually only be prescribed to women over 60 who are at high risk of osteoporosis. Para-thyroid hormone is reserved for women with a very high risk.

Hormone replacement therapy

HRT is the principal medical treatment available for troublesome menopausal symptoms and simply acts by replacing the hormones that are normally produced by the human ovary at physiological levels. Oestrogen is the main hormone and is either given alone or in combination with a progestogen, which should be given to all non-hysterectomized women. A third hormone, testosterone, can also be given in conjunction with oestrogen. Most HRT treatments come in prepared combinations, but it is important to understand the component parts.

Oestrogen

There are a variety of different types of oestrogen available, which can be given at varying doses and by different routes (Table 18.4). For the vast majority of women, the type and route of administration are not important and, provided an adequate dose of oestrogen is given, it is likely to be effective. However, there are some women who do not show an appropriate response and adjustment to a different type of oestrogen may be helpful. As with any treatment, the lowest possible dose should be used.

Different routes of oestrogen administration have different pharmacokinetic profiles. Non-oral routes, of which the transdermal route is the most widely used, avoid the first-pass effect and are considered more physiological as they release oestradiol into the circulation, rather than oestrone. Avoiding the first-pass effect reduces the impact on various metabolic parameters, such as the haemostatic and coagulation system, so seems a better option in women with a personal or relevant family history of venous thrombosis or known liver abnormalities.

Table 18.4 Different oestrogen and progestogen preparations used in HRT. All are available orally. Additional routes are listed.

Different oestrogens used in HRT	
Oestradiol (transdermal, gel, implant)	
Oestradiol valerate	
Conjugated equine oestrogens	
Oestrone sulphate	
Oestriol (vaginal only)	
Different progestogens used in HRT	
C-19 nortestosterone derivatives:	Norethisterone (transdermal)
	Levonorgestrel (transdermal, intrauterine)
C-21 progesterone derivatives:	Dydrogesterone
	Medroxyprogesterone acetate
	Cyproterone acetate (not available in UK)
C-17 derivatives:	Drospirenone
Progesterone:	Micronized progesterone (vaginal gel, pessary, suppository)

Non-oral routes tend to be more expensive and, for those women who need a progestogen, there can be logistical problems administering the progestogen component simultaneously. Subcutaneous implants tend to be reserved for women who do not respond to standard levels of oestrogen. They tend to be used more in younger women who have had a hysterectomy and their ovaries removed. They require a minor surgical procedure for insertion and this is repeated every six months or so. Oestradiol can accumulate so plasma levels should be monitored carefully before reinsertion. Implants also allow the addition of testosterone (see below under Testosterone).

Progesterone

Progesterone, produced by the corpus luteum, is an essential part of the normal menstrual cycle, transforming and consolidating the oestrogen-primed endometrium ready for pregnancy. Withdrawal of the progestogen after failure of the corpus luteum leads to endometrial shedding and menstrual bleeding. In HRT, progestogens (synthetic progesterones) are added for at least 10 days per calendar month to mimic the normal menstrual cycle and reduce the risk of endometrial hyperplasia and cancer associated with the prolonged use of unopposed oestrogen. They can either be given cyclically, mimicking the natural 28-day cycle and resulting in a regular withdrawal bleed, or continuously to prevent any bleeding, so-called 'no bleed' treatment. The latter is usually recommended for women who are clearly post-menopausal, while the former is usually prescribed for women who are perimenopausal. There are several different types of progestogen used in HRT (Table 18.4). Side effects are common, particularly in the first few months, and these may vary depending on the type and dose of progestogen used. Switching from one type of progestogen to another, or changing the route of administration can alleviate side effects in many cases. The advent of the levonorgestrel intrauterine system has allowed many women who could not tolerate any of the available progestogen combinations to continue HRT safely. Women who have been hysterectomized do not need a progestogen.

Testosterone

Fifty per cent of testosterone production in women is from the ovaries (the other 50 per cent is from peripheral fat stores and the adrenals). Testosterone production is not generally affected by natural menopause, although a decline in sex hormone-binding globulin (SHBG) may lead to a small rise in circulating free testosterone. However, women who undergo a surgical or chemoradiation-induced menopause may become relatively testosterone deficient. Symptoms can be hard to determine specifically, but classically are loss of libido, decreased sexual activity, fatigue and reduced feelings of physical well-being.

Risks and benefits of HRT

Ever since the introduction of HRT in the 1960s there have been concerns that the prolongation of exposure to natural hormones may have an adverse effect on the breast and other oestrogen-sensitive tissues. Yet, despite widespread use for several decades and numerous studies, there remains uncertainty and controversy about exactly what the risks are and how relevant they are to the majority of healthy post-menopausal women. What is clear is that HRT is an extremely effective treatment for menopausal symptoms and urogenital atrophy, is an effective treatment for osteoporosis and appears to have beneficial effects on the cardiovascular system if started around the time of menopause. The risks and benefits based on current grade A evidence are shown in Table 18.5.

The majority of women start HRT for the relief of menopausal symptoms. Oestrogen is very effective in relieving hot flushes with improvement usually noted within 4–6 weeks. HRT is far more effective than non-hormonal preparations, such as clonidine and SSRI.

The symptoms of vaginal and urogenital atrophy respond well to systemic or vaginal oestrogens. Vaginal or topical oestrogen preparations do not have any significant systemic activity so can usually be given safely in women in whom HRT is otherwise contraindicated. Treatment is usually commenced daily for 2 weeks then with the improvement in the vaginal epithelium can be reduced to once or twice weekly. This should be continued at a low maintenance dose for up to 12 months. Progestogens are not necessary with vaginal oestrogen preparations.

HRT is effective in the prevention of postmenopausal bone loss and osteoporotic fractures at the spine and hip. Thus, women taking HRT for symptom relief will derive benefit as far as their bones are concerned. However, because of uncertainty about its long-term safety, the regulatory authorities

Table 18.5   Risks, benefits and uncertainties of HRT based on grade A evidence

Benefits	Risks	Uncertainties
Vasomotor symptoms	Breast cancer	Cardiovascular disease and stroke
Urogenital symptoms and sexual function	VTE	Alzheimer's
Stroke	Endometrial cancer	Ovarian cancer
Osteoporosis		
Colon cancer		

From British Menopause Society Consensus Statement. Available from: www.thebms.org.uk.

currently advise that HRT should not be used as a first-line treatment for osteoporosis prevention as the potential risks outweigh the benefits. However, they also emphasize that HRT is the most appropriate treatment for osteoporosis prevention in women with premature ovarian failure under the age of 50 and for women in whom the standard osteoporosis treatments are not tolerated or are unsuitable.

While there is convincing evidence that HRT started around the menopause does have a protective effect against cardiovascular disease, this is not an indication for considering HRT. Similarly, despite consistent evidence of reduced rates of colon cancer with HRT, this is not considered an indication.

Risks of HRT

Breast cancer

Controversy continues to surround the true effect of HRT on breast cancer risk. Part of the continuing uncertainty exists because most of the studies have been observational and such studies can only suggest an association with a factor (in this case HRT), they do not prove a true cause and effect. A large meta-analysis of observational studies published in 1997 probably still provides us with the best information. This stated that if HRT was used for less than five years in the early post-menopause it does not appear to increase breast cancer risk. Thereafter, there does appear to be a small increase in risk of 1.35 (95 per cent confidence interval, 1.20–1.49). In absolute numbers, this equates to four extra breast cancer cases per 1000 women who use HRT from the age of 50 for five years (Figure 18.7). The magnitude of risk appears to be similar to that associated with late natural menopause (2.3 per cent

compared with 2.8 per cent per year, respectively) and increases with years of exposure. Women who start HRT early for premature menopause do not show this effect, suggesting that it may be the lifetime sex hormone exposure that is relevant. More recently, a large randomized trial on HRT (the Women's Health Initiative (WHI)), reported a broadly similar risk to that seen in the epidemiological studies for combined oestrogen and progestogen treatment after five years, but also found no increase in risk over seven years with oestrogen-only treatment. Thus, the increase in risk seems to be more associated with the progestogen component. Furthermore, a recent French study has suggested that certain types of progestogen may be associated with lower risks than others.

In summary, otherwise healthy postmenopausal women in their late 40s and 50s wishing to take HRT should be reassured that the overall risk of developing breast cancer in the first few years as a result of their HRT is small. If they take oestrogen alone, that risk is probably even lower. Breast cancer is a multifactorial disease and overall other personal risk factors, such as family history, are likely to be more important predictive factors.

Endometrial cancer

Unopposed oestrogen replacement therapy increases endometrial cancer risk which is why all non-hysterctomized women should also receive a progestogen. These are usually given cyclically to mimic the natural menstrual cycle. This gives a monthly withdrawal bleed, but once a woman is clearly postmenopausal, she should be switched to a continuous combined (no bleed) regimen. Any abnormal bleeding on HRT should be investigated,

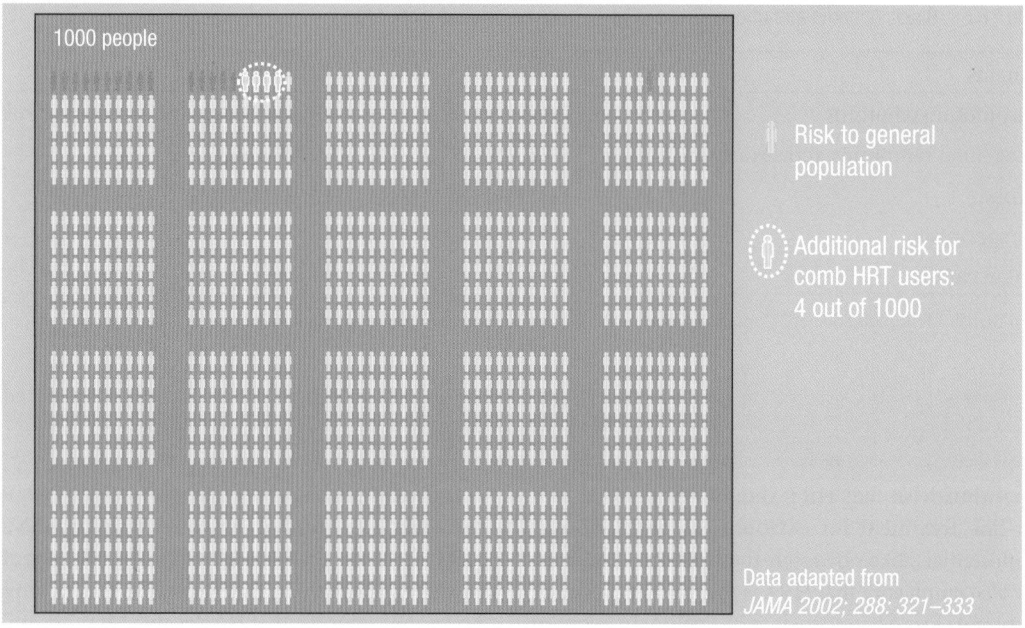

Figure 18.7 Schematic representation of the risk for postmenopausal women (mean age 63 years) developing breast cancer over a five-year period and how this would be influenced by taking HRT. The background risk is 15/1000 and if all these women took HRT for those five years an extra four would develop breast cancer. Data adapted from Women's Health Initiative Randomized Controlled Trial. *Journal of the American Medical Association* 2002; **288**: 321–33.

although the likelihood of underlying malignancy is low.

Ovarian cancer

Most of the limited data relate to oestrogen alone and suggest a small increase in risk with very long term (>10 years) treatment. This increase does not seem apparent with combined therapy.

Venous thromboembolism

HRT increases the risk of venous thromboembolism (VTE) two-fold, with the highest risk occurring in the first year of use. The background risk of VTE in women over 50 years not taking HRT is small (1.7/1000), so the overall impact of this increase is very low. However, the background risk is significantly increased in women who smoke, are obese, have an underlying thrombophilia such as Factor V Leiden or who have previously suffered a VTE. Transdermal HRT has less impact on haemostatic mechanisms and appears to be associated with a lower risk of VTE even in women with a thrombophilia, and thus may be the treatment of choice in this group.

Coronary heart disease

From the data discussed earlier, it is clear there is a conflict between large-scale epidemiological studies which have consistently shown that oestrogens appears to have a protective effect on CHD and the more recent randomized trials which suggest a possible adverse effect. Subsequent detailed analysis of these and other data suggest that timing of the introduction of oestrogen may be critical. For women starting HRT shortly after menopause, there may well be a protective effect on CHD, and this particularly appears to be the case for women undergoing premature menopause. However, in women many years past the menopause, starting HRT may have a detrimental effect. HRT should not be used specifically for cardiovascular disease protection.

Stroke

Small increases in the risk of stroke with both oestrogen-only and combined oestrogen and progestogen were reported in the WHI study, although there was a significant age effect, with a relatively high risk in older women and no reported increase in the 50–59-age group. In general, the data suggests a trend towards a small increased incidence of stroke with HRT, and HRT should not be initiated for women over the age of 60, or those who have strong risk factors for stroke or cardiovascular disease risk without carefully weighing up the potential risks against any potential benefits.

Practical considerations for prescribing HRT

HRT is only one option for dealing with menopausal symptoms and other options can be considered. Yet, despite the recent controversies, HRT remains the clinically most effective and cost-effective strategy for women with menopausal symptoms. For the majority of healthy symptomatic menopausal women, the potential benefits will outweigh any small risks. However, like all treatments, the risks and benefits should be weighed up individually with the patient before starting treatment. The absolute and relative contraindications are listed in Table 18.6. Women with relative contraindications may still be suitable for HRT, but would benefit from specialist assessment and possibly further investigations. For example, a woman with a past history of VTE should not be given HRT until an underlying thrombophilia has been excluded.

Table 18.6   Absolute and relative contraindications to taking HRT

Absolute	Suspected pregnancy
	Breast cancer
	Endometrial cancer
	Active liver disease
	Uncontrolled hypertension
	Known VTE
	Known thrombophilia (e.g. Factor V leiden)
	Otosclerosis
Relative	Uninvestigated abnormal bleeding
	Large uterine fibroids
	Past history of benign breast disease
	Unconfirmed personal history or a strong family history of VTE
	Chronic stable liver disease
	Migraine with aura

Selecting which HRT regimen is a matter for the individual prescriber. If there are specific special circumstances, then a particular type or route of administration may be most appropriate. Follow up should be arranged after about three months to check the treatment's effectiveness and any persistent side effects. There are over 80 preparations available, but the majority of women respond well to whatever treatment they are given. Treatment should be started at the lowest appropriate dose and can be increased if there is no symptomatic improvement after a few months. Side effects from the reintroduction of oestrogen and progesterone may be common particularly if it has been several years since the menopause. Common side effects are listed in Table 18.7. Oestrogen-related side effects are usually dose related and settle within a few weeks. Progestogenic side effects are more troublesome and often resemble premenstrual symptoms. If persistent, then a change in progestogen type may be helpful (Table 18.4).

Table 18.7   Common side effects with HRT

Oestrogen related	Progestogen related
Fluid retention	Fluid retention
Nausea	Breast tenderness
Headaches	Headaches
Breast enlargement	Acne
Leg cramps	Mood swings
Dyspepsia	Depression
	Irritability
	Bloating
	Constipation
	Increased appetite

The duration of HRT use depends on the individual circumstances and indication for taking it. The 'average' menopausal woman in her early 50s will probably only take it for two or three years, but there is no reason why she should not take it for longer if indicated. The MHRA recommend taking 'the minimum effective dose' of HRT for the 'shortest duration' without defining any specific length of time. Based on other recommendations, this has generally been interpreted as about five years, although in reality most women do not take it that long. However, treatment can be continued for longer in women with persistent troublesome symptoms that adversely affect their quality of life. The exception to these recommendations is women who have undergone a premature menopause. In this group, the risk/benefit balance is strongly in favour of them taking HRT at least up until the age of 50 as a true physiological replacement.

Once stabilized on treatment, women should be reviewed every six months or so. Their individual risk of VTE, stroke and breast cancer should be appraised regularly and balanced against the benefits they are gaining from the treatment. For the majority of women, the overall increase in any risk will be small and some women will opt to continue taking HRT for its benefits well into their 60s. Women on HRT should continue to participate in the national screening programmes for breast, cervical and colorectal cancer. There is no indication for more frequent assessments or for regular pelvic examinations unless there is unscheduled bleeding or another clinical development. Stopping HRT should be done gradually, reducing the dose to avoid rebound symptoms. At the same time, positive lifestyle factors should be emphasized, such as diet and regular exercise. Vaginal oestrogens can be added in if troublesome genitourinary symptoms persist.

While a truly menopausal woman cannot conceive, defining when that moment has occurred is extremely difficult. Thus contraception should be continued until two years after the last period in women under 50 and one year in women over 50. HRT itself is not a contraceptive and serum FSH levels are not particularly reliable on HRT. Condoms will reduce the incidence of sexually transmitted infections (STI), particularly for those in new relationships. The levonegestrel intrauterine system (IUS) is particularly useful in this age group as the device provides ongoing contraception and endometrial protection allowing oestrogen to be added when symptoms develop.

New developments

There is ongoing research into development of the ideal postmenopausal treatment that will control symptoms, prevent bone loss, reduce cardiovascular disease risk, but at the same time not increase risks of breast cancer, endometrial cancer and VTE. To this end, a new generation of selective tissue receptor modulators are being developed which will have selective action against oestrogen, progesterone and testosterone receptors. Currently, raloxifene is the only SERM commercially available. Raloxifene is a benzothiphene and is closely related to tamoxifen. It acts by locking into the oestrogen receptors, but as it does so its side chain deactivates one of the activation functions of the receptor. This specific action only occurs in certain tissues, such as the breast and endometrium. In other tissues, such as the skeleton, the side arm does not deactivate the receptor and raloxifene behaves like an oestrogen. At present, these products do not relieve menopausal symptoms so are primarily restricted for women at risk of osteoporosis.

Key Points

- The menopause is a hormonal milestone that occurs in all women and provides an opportunity to identify specific risks and build for a healthy future. The mean age of onset is around 51–52 years.
- The central change is a dramatic fall in the amount of circulating oestrogen.
- Premature menopause should be considered as a diagnosis in any women under 45 with prolonged (>6 months) amenorrhoea.
- Oestrogen has far-ranging effects throughout the body.
- Hormone replacement is a very effective treatment for menopausal symptoms but is only one option.
- HRT will also stop bone loss after menopause and reduce the risk of fracture.
- As with any treatment, there are some risks with HRT that should be weighed up with the patient before starting HRT.
- For the majority of symptomatic postmenopausal women, the benefits of taking HRT will outweigh any small risks but this should be assessed individually.
- HRT consist of two hormones:
  - Oestrogen is the main one and should be prescribed at the lowest effective dose. Different routes may be useful in some medical conditions.
  - Progestogens are needed in all women with an intact uterus. There are a variety of types which can either be given cyclically or continuously.
- There are a large number of alternative preparations available for menopausal symptoms, but most of them have very little supportive or safety data.

CASE HISTORY

Mrs JS is a generally fit 53-year-old primary school teacher who presents with troublesome hot flushes, night sweats and generalized tiredness over the last six months. Her menstrual cycle has become erratic, sometimes missing a month, but her bleeding is not heavy. On close questioning she is sleeping badly, waking up soaking wet several times a night. She is permanently tired and irritable and on several occasions has lost her temper in the classroom which is very uncharacteristic. She has tried several over-the-counter preparations without much benefit. She has thought about HRT, but is concerned because her mother had breast cancer at the age of 64. Her mother is still alive and well, but suffers with osteoporosis. Mrs JS has no other significant history and is up to date with her smears and mammograms. She is married and is sexually active, although at present they are sleeping separately because of her disturbed sleep.

Discussion

Mrs JS is presenting with classical menopausal symptoms. Whether the tiredness and irritability is a direct effect of the menopause or secondary to her poor sleep is debatable, but either way her symptoms are significantly affecting her quality of life. She would be a good candidate for HRT, but is concerned about the potential risk of breast cancer. Although there is a family history, this is not deemed a significant risk, thus Mrs JS's personal risk is no greater than anyone else's.

Treatment

Mrs JS still has a uterus so she will need combined HRT and as she is still having a menstrual cycle this would be best given as a sequential product to give a monthly withdrawal bleed. Any one of a variety of products would be suitable. Usually, a low-dose (1 mg) oral preparation would be used first with review at three months. If the symptoms were not controlled, then the dose could be increased. Any side effects should be assessed at that point and if necessary a different preparation prescribed. A full discussion should be had with her regarding the potential benefits and risks of HRT, but she can be reassured that the risks for her are very small and outweighed by the potential benefits. She should be encouraged to continue with normal mammographic screening and self breast examination, but there is no need for any more frequent assessments. In view of her family history of osteoporosis, a DEXA bone scan would be helpful. This will give her an indication of her long-term risk. Regardless of the result, she should be informed that managing and preventing osteoporosis is a lifelong strategy. She can be reassured that while taking HRT she is getting preservation of her bone density. She should aim to take regular weight bearing exercise for at least 20 minutes three times/ week and have a balanced diet with plenty of calcium. If her calcium intake is less than 800 mg/day she should take supplementation. A repeat bone scan in three to five years would be advisable. If the T score shows osteopenia (between −1.5 and −2.5) then she may require ongoing treatment with a bisphosphonate when she eventually stops her HRT.

However, further work is ongoing with similar preparations, in combination with small amounts of oestrogen, which from initial studies appear promising.

There is also renewed interest in the cause of hot flushes and the development of some newer drugs that may act on the serotonin pathway and reduce vasomotor symptoms.

Additional reading

Al-Azzawi F, Barlow D, Hillard T *et al*. Prevention and treatment of osteoporosis in women. British Menopause Society Consensus Statement. *Menopause International* 2007; **13**: 178–81. Available from: www.thebms.org.uk/statements.php.

Basson R, Berman J, Burnett A *et al*. Report of the international consensus development conference on female sexual dysfunction: definitions and classifications. Journal of Urology 2000; **163**: 888–93.

Birkhauser MH, Panay N, Archer DF *et al*. Updated recommendations for hormone replacement therapy in the peri- and postmenopause. *Climacteric* 2008; **11**: 108–23.

Medicines and Healthcare Products Regulatory Agency and Commission on Human Medicines. Hormone replacement therapy: updated advice. *Drug Safety Update* 2007; **1**: 2–5.

National Institute for Health and Clinical Excellence. Alendronate, etidronate, risedronate, raloxifene and strontium ranelate for the primary prevention of osteoporotic fragility fractures in postmenopausal women. TA161, October 2008. Available from: www.nice.org.

NIH Consensus Development Panel on Osteoporosis Prevention, Diagnosis and Therapy. *Journal of the American Medical Association* 2001; **285**: 785–95.

Panay N, Rees M. Alternatives to HRT for the management of symptoms of the menopause (SAC Opinion Paper 6). Available from: www.rcog.org.uk/womens-health/clinical-guidance/alternatives-hrt-management-symptoms-menopause.

Poole KES, Compston JE. Osteoporosis and it management. *British Medical Journal* 2006; **333**: 1251–6.

Rees M, Stevenson J, Hope S *et al. Management of the menopause*. London: British Menopause Society and RSM Press, 2009.

Rymer J, Morris EP. Extracts from 'Clinical Evidence': menopausal symptoms. *British Medical Journal* 2000; **321**: 1516–19.

Speroff L, Glass RH, Kase NG. *Clinical gynecologic endocrinology and infertility*. Baltimore, MD: Williams & Wilkins, 1990: 121–64.

Suckling J, Lethaby A, Kennedy R. Local oestrogen for vaginal atrophy in postmenopausal women. *Cochrane Database of Systematic Reviews* 2006; (**4**): CD001500.

Writing Group for the Women's Health Initiative Investigators. Risks and benefits of estrogen plus progestin in healthy postmenopausal women. Principal results from the Women's Health Initiative Randomized Controlled Trial. *Journal of the American Medical Association* 2002; **288**: 321–33.

CHAPTER 19

PSYCHOSOCIAL AND ETHICAL ASPECTS OF GYNAECOLOGY

OVERVIEW

In gynaecology, the personal nature of the clinical problems makes it crucial to appreciate the social, cultural and psychological context in which they are presented. It is important to be aware that presented symptoms may sometimes only be a key to larger concerns or events occurring in that individual's life.

All women face significant life events and decisions that are intimately involved with their gendered physiology and body. Gynaecologists are expected to understand these, provide advice that is evidence-based and also respect individuals' values and lifestyle.

It is not uncommon to see physical symptoms that have no demonstrable organic pathology, such as dyspareunia (pain with intercourse) or dysmenorrhoea (painful periods). Women also suffer psychological symptoms as a response to disease (e.g. infertility or cancer).

The nature of gynaecological problems means that sexual and relationship problems are inevitably entwined and there are new challenges and issues at every stage of the reproductive life cycle.

Puberty

Adolescence is defined by the pubertal transition, when young people undergo intense physical growth and often feel self-conscious about their changing bodies. Girls will be dealing with menstruation and trying to cope with the pressures of school, peers and new feelings and experiences. Teenagers are more likely to engage in high-risk sexual behaviour, making them vulnerable to unplanned pregnancies and sexually transmitted infections.

Understandably, parents may attend consultations with young women. Indeed, it may be relevant if they do not attend, or if they attend and do not allow their daughter some private time with a doctor or nurse. Without confidential time, it may not be appropriate, or possible, to discuss certain topics (such as contraception or home circumstances) even when

these may be relevant and important. It is important to elicit the history from the patient herself and not through a third party (i.e. the parent or boyfriend).

Competence is not determined by age but is function-specific. Increasingly, there is medical awareness of this, though sometimes we become desensitized to the issues involved. Guidelines on competence in under-16s and the Fraser Guidelines (Box 19.1) are important to understand. Difficult decisions may otherwise be handed back to young patients as if they were adults without realizing that they may not have an adequate support structure to make those decisions or to stick to certain management plans. For example, a 15-year-old attending an early pregnancy unit for follow up for a possible ectopic pregnancy may not have disclosed that she is pregnant to anyone else. She may be skipping classes to attend appointments, placing more stress on herself. She may

> **Box 19.1 The Fraser Guidelines for competency**
>
> A doctor is able to give contraceptive treatment or advice to a person under the age of 16 years provided:
>
> - the patient is mature enough to understand the advice given and its implications;
> - the patient is likely to begin and continue to have sex with or without advice/contraception;
> - the practitioner has made attempts to advise the patient to notify a suitable adult;
> - the patient's health will suffer without treatment or advice.

not be able to disclose symptoms suggestive of rupture to her family, therefore delaying access to prompt treatment.

Unwanted pregnancy

Unplanned and unwanted pregnancies are common, leading to an annual abortion rate of around 18.5 per 1000 women. Women struggle with the decision to continue or end an unplanned pregnancy, considering their own circumstances and the opinions of their partner, family, friends, doctors and the general public. A pregnancy can change from wanted to unwanted (and vice versa) through the reactions of others or external economic pressure. In some instances, women may be thrilled and welcome an unexpected pregnancy. In other cases, women with an initially much wanted pregnancy may later seek termination due to fetal abnormality or a threat to personal health.

Most women feel relief and do not regret a decision to terminate pregnancy. Some may experience guilt, shame and embarrassment which can be worsened by unsympathetic health professionals. Fearing disapproval, women may not reveal what happened or their emotions to anyone, becoming isolated and burdened with this 'secret'. The experience can be especially difficult to cope with for women who themselves have negative attitudes against abortion and yet felt they had no choice when making the decision.

Women who are coping with a continuing unwanted pregnancy are more likely to become stressed and depressed as the pregnancy progresses. Women have poorer psychological outcomes if their partner is unsupportive or rejects the pregnancy, and there may be worse outcomes for children too, especially if termination has been sought and refused.

Early pregnancy loss

A substantial minority of all pregnancies end spontaneously in the first trimester or present as an ectopic, possibly even before the woman is aware that she is pregnant. The initial diagnosis of early pregnancy loss may involve several appointments and scans causing much anxiety. The sense of hopelessness, while little can be done except wait for days or weeks, can be emotionally draining – not only for the woman but also her partner, family or friends. A spontaneous miscarriage can be a traumatic experience involving emergency admission to A&E and significant bleeding and pain. There are added stresses of having to deal with the management and interventions for delayed or incomplete miscarriages.

When a diagnosis of miscarriage is made, the emotional reactions can range between denial, guilt, a sense of failure, anger and grief. Early loss does not draw in the same social support and rituals which accompany the death of any loved person and there may be an inability to mourn or grieve.

As spontaneous miscarriages are largely related to sporadic chromosomal anomalies, the investigations performed are often negative, providing little consolation as there is nothing to change or treat next time. Grief and anxiety following an early loss can be carried into the next pregnancy or result in a need to be 'in control'. Recurrent early losses can have even more profound implications for the woman's view of herself and her body. There may be pressures from the partner, fear of breakdown of relationships as well as the 'biological clock' ticking.

The life-threatening nature of ectopic pregnancy creates another dimension to the loss. Women may lose their Fallopian tube or ovary as part of treatment and sterility is a possible outcome.

Premenstrual problems

Between 2 and 10 per cent of women experience severe premenstrual symptoms that interfere with their daily life and relationships with others. Individual differences in beliefs and coping strategies may lead to women experiencing cyclic physiological changes in the premenstrual phase in ways that exacerbate emotional reactions.

Psychosocial factors have been implicated in the aetiology of premenstrual syndrome. These include stressful life events, relationship dissatisfaction and attribution of negative moods to the menstrual cycle. Thoughts such as 'I can't cope' or 'If I'm not in control people will not like me' can create anxiety and lead to heightened responses and emotional lability.

Some feminists think that the premenstrual phase gives women an insight into valid feelings which they should heed and attend to in the calmer times. The psychological influences in premenstrual syndrome have been well recognized and a biopsychosocial approach is used, with management involving cognitive behavioural therapy.

Subfertility and infertility

Difficulty or failure to conceive is very stressful with repeated cycles of hope and disappointment. In seeking help for infertility, a woman not only has to expose her body but also her relationship and intimate self with strangers. She enters an unfamiliar clinical world. The initial high levels of motivation may overcome the negatives. With increasing intrusions, drugs and procedures, the optimism fades and dissatisfaction and low tolerance for the processes can ensue. Life centres around the desire to have a baby. The setbacks may result in partners blaming each other and becoming frustrated and guilty.

Following an unsuccessful attempt to conceive a couple can be left deeply wounded. The natural right to found a family has been denied. The acceptance of this can be difficult and complicated. The dream of identity as a mother or father is shattered. Indeed, the loss of ability to present grandchildren, nieces and nephews or cousins to the extended family affects many others too. The image of the child and family (that has been denied) must be mourned. As the majority of assisted conception patients do not have children, counselling about the possibility, or preparedness, for moving on should start with the onset of investigation and treatment. Counselling services exist within assisted conception units to help with decision-making, the stresses of the process and the emotions surrounding failure, giving up and resolution.

Body image

Over millennia, great importance has been placed on women's external appearance. Abnormal attitudes to body shape, and consequent eating disorders, can affect menstrual cycles. Sometimes women adopt unusual practices to enhance their appearance. Currently, this includes cosmetic surgery which has extended into the gynaecological arena with concepts such as restoring virginity, or creating a 'designer vagina'.

Women may attend clinics to obtain reassurance about their normality. It is important not to use language or gaze that makes them more self-conscious. In a clinical environment, what we see as clinical signs (e.g. obesity, hirsutism) can exacerbate negative body awareness and low self-esteem. Joking, flirting or sexualized comments during a consultation are considered inappropriate or even serious professional misconduct.

Chronic pelvic pain

Chronic pelvic pain is a common symptom presenting to general practitioners, genitourinary medicine and gynaecology clinics. It can be a challenging condition for women and their clinicians. Doctors concentrate on diagnosing or ruling out organic pathology (such as endometriosis or pelvic infection/adhesions) and naturally 'medicalize' presentations when formulating a differential diagnosis. Therefore, when no recognizable pathology is found, which is often, it becomes tricky to backtrack and start to explore the psychological aspects. This approach can make patients feel their pain is being dismissed as merely being 'in their head'.

It is important to address and explore psychosocial factors from the first consultation. This should be as part of the normal 'routine' history. Much can be revealed from the past medical, family and social history. Self-monitoring and heightened awareness of pain are particularly apparent in women who have a past history of pelvic pathology, obstetric complications and a family history of pelvic disease. Consulting behaviour is also heavily influenced by messages from family members about the significance of symptoms. Previous adverse events, such as child abuse, violence or rape may play a part. Clinicians must become skilled, sympathetic and comfortable in such psychosocial questioning and in handling tears or upsetting answers.

Menopause

Though there are biological and physiological changes during the climacteric period leading to the menopause, it is essentially a natural life process. The range of psychological reactions to this aspect of reproductive ageing can range from relief to dread.

The two greatest factors regarding the subjective experience of menopause are:

- what women believe and anticipate about the menopause – which has a direct bearing on how they experience it;
- the clear link between lifestyle factors, such as body mass index, exercise and smoking, and the frequency and severity of symptoms.

Social scientists believe that a woman's attitude towards the menopause directly influences the sort of experience she has. This can also be a time of major life changes: children leaving home, retirement of one or both partners, death or disability of parents or spouse. The change of lifestyle with additional distracting symptoms, such as hot flushes, poor sleep and vaginal dryness, can cause irritability and low mood.

Though hormone replacement therapy (HRT) can help with vasomotor symptoms, it is not a cure-all for the other changes or symptoms women experience. Therefore, it is important to explore reasons for using HRT and expectations of it.

Cancer

The diagnosis of a gynaecological cancer causes a woman to face the possibility of mortality but, in addition, may strike at her sexuality and fertility. The uterus, ovaries and breasts are all symbols of a woman's fertility. The threat of losing them as a result of disease or treatment can cause a woman to question her identity and impact her sexual function and relationships. Women who have not completed their family may face the possibility of losing their fertility as part of the battle against the disease.

Psychosexual disorders

About 43 per cent of women report experiencing sexual difficulties. Despite the prevalence of these problems, they are presented only infrequently as such to clinicians. Often, they are presented indirectly along with other complaints such as pelvic pain, menstrual problems and dissatisfaction with contraception. The underlying problems are easily overlooked as patients attend repeatedly at different services with unsatisfactory consultations.

Sexual response cycle

To appreciate this group of gynaecological problems, it is important to be familiar with normal female sexual response. Traditionally, the sexual response cycle seen involves four phases:

1 Desire
2 Arousal
3 Orgasm
4 Resolution

Though this marks out the physiological processes, it does not provide an adequate appreciation of the psychological overlay of the sexual response. It is also based on a traditional and heterosexual model where it is assumed that penetration and orgasm are the ultimate goals rather than self-satisfaction or bonding and intimacy.

Recent definitions acknowledge the importance of the sexual relationship, placing emotional and sexual satisfaction as equally important. There is an appreciation that the four phases are not a linear progression but are likely to overlap.

Classification of sexual disorders

The *Diagnostic and statistical manual of mental disorders IV* of the American Psychiatric Association (DSM-IV) classifies sexual dysfunction into four categories (Box 19.2).

Sexual desire disorders

Physiological factors, such as the menopause and depression, are known to affect sexual desire. However, sexual desire disorders are heavily influenced by psychological factors.

> **Box 19.2 DSM-IV Classification of female sexual dysfunction**
>
> 1 Sexual desire disorders
> 2 Hypoactive sexual desire disorder
> 3 Sexual aversion disorder
> 4 Sexual arousal disorder
> 5 Orgasmic disorder
> 6 Sexual pain disorders

Early negative experiences surrounding culture, loss and previous relationships can result in negative feelings that lead to avoidance of sexual intimacy. These emotions may include guilt, shame and embarrassment. Unrealistic expectations that sexual desire is a spontaneous response may create anticipatory anxiety surrounding intimacy. In some situations, underlying problems in the relationship are relevant (e.g. unequal power or infidelity).

Sexual arousal disorders

This can be an inability to achieve either physiological or subjective arousal. The physical changes of vaginal lubrication and pelvic congestion, associated with arousal, can occur without the ability to access the subjective experience of pleasure. Likewise, subjective arousal can be met with a lack of physical changes causing much frustration. Mental disengagement and lack of awareness of the sensations of arousal can also contribute.

Orgasmic disorders

Failure to achieve orgasm (anorgasmia) is more common in younger women, suggesting that sexual response is a learned response – often achieved through masturbation, or experimentation with a trusted partner. This could be a constant problem or one that arises with a specific partner.

Personal factors, such as the inability to lose control and cultural reasons surrounding the female enjoyment of intercourse can all be factors surrounding anorgasmia. Penetrative intercourse alone is not sufficient to achieve orgasm in most women. Failure to communicate her wishes during intercourse can lead to a woman's dissatisfaction and failure to achieve orgasm.

Sexual pain disorders

Vaginismus

This is defined as the persistent or recurrent difficulties of a woman to allow vaginal entry of any object, despite her expressed wish to do so. There is involuntary contraction of pelvic muscles with anticipation, fear or experience of pain.

It can arise as a conditioned response to adverse physical or psychological experiences in the past. Previous traumatic sexual experiences can make pelvic examination and intimate sexual contact distressing and painful. Painful childbirth and previous gynaecological procedures or examinations may have created anxiety around any intimate contact.

Vulval vestibulitis

This is characterized by pain at the introitus on penetration leading to tenderness and erythema. After dermatological conditions, such as lichen sclerosus, psoriasis and dermatoses, have been ruled out, this diagnosis is to be considered. Patients may find it reassuring when this is explained and acknowledged. The recognition of this pain being valid can in itself be therapeutic to women.

Considering the very intimate and delicate nature of these problems, it is easy to see how women tend not to reveal the true nature of their complaints. Therefore, it can easily be overlooked when assessing a woman's symptoms. Confident, sensitive and routine asking about sexual function (without prurience) can reduce the patient's embarrassment of revealing these problems to a clinician.

Adverse experiences and abuse

Women and children are vulnerable to specific adverse experiences and abuse due to their gender and age. As we enter the psychological world of patients we may stumble across painful, hidden aspects of their past or current lives. Sometimes these matters will have a bearing on their symptoms, diagnosis, coping mechanisms or ability to follow medical advice. Sometimes they will not be relevant.

Due to stigma, shame and unhelpful stereotypes, many patients will not reveal or discuss bad or painful experiences unless they have picked up cues from the clinician that they will not be dismissed or judged. Sensitive questioning may reveal past or current vulnerability and doctors must be ready to listen, sympathize and make relevant referrals to agencies with expertise (whether professional, voluntary sector or self-help groups).

A few issues particularly pertinent to gynaecology are discussed below.

Adverse childhood experiences

Many patients will have had adverse circumstances in their childhood such as neglect, abandonment, physical, sexual or psychological abuse. They may have experienced early bereavement or had a disrupted family life. Their carers may have struggled with poverty, disability, mental illness, violence, criminality, alcohol or substance misuse. Some children may have been carers for parents or siblings. Asking about early sexual experiences or unwanted sexual attention may reveal a history of child sexual abuse. Adverse childhood experiences have lifetime effects and colour reactions to personal illness.

Domestic violence

Domestic violence is an underreported hidden crime. About one in four women during their lifetime, and one in ten in current relationships, experience physical or emotional abuse from a current or former partner. Intimate partner violence is not confined to certain ages, racial backgrounds or socioeconomic groups. As part of the abuse, women may be systematically isolated from their family and friends. Their lives, clothes, food and whereabouts can be jealously controlled and they are undermined, insulted and blamed for provoking the abuse. The greatest danger is at, or after, the end of a relationship. In the UK, over two women a week are killed by an ex- or current partner. It is crucial for medical professionals to learn to identify and deal appropriately with domestic violence.

The presentation of domestic abuse is only rarely as an emergency. Abuse presents more insidiously, sometimes with odd symptoms, or chronic pain or an unusual history. The partners may be obviously aggressive or overly solicitous. Women may attend late for a check-up for a miscarriage after a 'fall', miss appointments or discharge themselves against medical advice. It is therefore wise to have a dose of suspicion in all consultations and ask direct questions about domestic circumstances and safety in a routine way.

Sexual assault in the context of domestic violence can be a terrifying experience, accounting for over half of UK rapes. It is an intimate violation from someone who had been trusted and given emotional investment. To compound this, many women feel that they cannot say no in the context of marriage. Women experiencing domestic violence are at risk of repeat victimization and their past history can reveal sexual abuse and previous violent relationships.

Rape

Rape is the penetration of the vagina, anus or mouth with a penis in the absence of consent. Though stranger rape and date rape are often the images that come to mind, about half of women raped know the perpetrator. There is a hesitancy to disclose rape for several reasons: fear of not being believed, the stigma of being a victim, self-blame and shame. As a result, only half of women disclose their rape to anyone. The clinician's role in the care of women is physical, forensic and psychological:

- **Physical:** The immediate clinical concerns are the treatment of any sustained injuries, contraceptive cover, exclusion of pregnancy and prevention, or treatment, of infections (e.g. post-exposure HIV (human immunodeficiency virus) prophylaxis).

- **Forensic:** It is a clinician's duty to document meticulously and accurately the patient's account of the story and any injuries sustained. There are genital injuries to document in less than 25 per cent of cases. Sometimes lacerations and bruises elsewhere on the body may provide evidence of a struggle. Specialist forensic sampling may be needed to obtain DNA of the assailant.

- **Psychological:** The response to rape can be varied. Women may have problems establishing new relationships. If the assailant was an acquaintance or relative, she may fear to trust her own judgement. There may be avoidance behaviour, such as avoiding being alone. Rape trauma syndrome has been described as a form of post-traumatic disorder resulting in physical, psychological and behavioural changes.

Sexual violence and torture

Some women, particularly those who have been trafficked, have been forced to work as prostitutes in the sex industry. Increasingly, we see women in the UK who have come from other countries and experienced sexual violence as a weapon of war. Rape is used to control and degrade and is often used as a form of torture with both men and women. Certain ideas are then attached to the sexual violence resulting in the victim having a changed opinion on her self-worth, sexuality and fertility. Asylum seekers and refugees who flee their homelands due to chaos and unrest struggle to establish an identity. They may not be able to speak about their experiences.

Female genital mutilation and harmful traditional practices

Not uncommonly, women can be victims of cultural and traditional community practices such as female genital mutilation (FGM), forced marriages and so-called 'honour killings'. These can present themselves in far more complex ways. It is important to recognize that there are common basic human rights the world over, while recognizing cultural differences and reacting to patients' individual concerns.

Handling disclosures

Sometimes, women make their first disclosure of their experiences to a clinician during a consultation. Disclosure is a complicated process, with mental and social barriers, in the groups of women discussed. They may find it more acceptable to seek attention to talk about pain and disruptive menstrual periods rather than tell the whole story, and expose their vulnerability and need for support.

The clinician's reaction may then affect how they go on to deal with the situation. Doctors' instincts can be to take a paternalistic stance and tell the patient what to do next. However, in view of the loss of control that previous events represent, it is important to ensure that women continue to have some control over their lives.

Witnessing by a sympathetic clinician may be all that is required; in both senses of (1) being empathetic and stating 'what was done to you was wrong' and (2) legally, in terms of written documentation. Validation during a medical consultation can be helpful in encouraging the woman to carry that power into her own situation and enable her to make changes in her life (e.g. making a safety plan, leaving her abusive partner, finding a healing ritual or taking legal action

against a sexual assailant). A clumsy response may only reinforce or repeat the victimization.

Women's concerns about safety must always be heeded. They may be concerned about their physical safety, or how their information is handled. Safety and confidentiality are paramount. The key question to ask is 'are you safe to go home?'.

Summary

There are many psychosocial aspects in gynaecology to learn about in addition to the medical and surgical disorders. The key skill to learn is thorough and sensitive history taking. A positive and sympathetic attitude to women has to be cultivated. The areas relating to psychological issues in gynaecology covered above are not exhaustive. In addition, there are other psychological challenges in obstetrics – such as tokophobia (a pathological fear of childbirth), stillbirth, post-natal depression and traumatic childbirth.

We now move on to the legal and ethical frameworks in which medicine is practised, and understanding those aspects specifically relating to gynaecology.

Ethics in gynaecology

Ethics is the science of morals, the branch of philosophy that is concerned with human character and conduct. Therefore, any action within the doctor–patient relationship will have an ethical dimension.

We all need to consider ethics for several reasons:

- To decide if an action is right or wrong
- To guide us in the future when a dilemma occurs
- To know the extent of our professional obligations
- For society to set boundaries of unacceptable behaviour through guidelines or laws.

There are frameworks that exist when analysing ethical dilemmas (Box 19.3). At first glance, these frameworks can seem academic, mutually incompatible or even irrelevant. Surely, doctors have good morals and values and instinctively make the right decisions?

Although only a tiny minority of doctors are ever struck off for serious professional misconduct, correct professional attributes need to be learned and practised. It is important to recognize the 'queasy feeling' that something is not right. We might face this feeling as students witnessing unprofessional behaviour, or as qualified doctors performing procedures beyond our competence, when we are desperate to please a sick or pleading patient, or when we receive our first complaint. It is when dealing with such situations that we realize that the distinction between right and wrong may not be so clear. Recognizing one's own limitations and asking appropriately for help are ethical qualities.

All medical actions, however trivial or exotic, have a clinical, legal and ethical dimension. Doctors have to bring medical knowledge and clinical expertise to bear on the patient's problem. Often, that is straightforward, but sometimes not.

Box 19.3 Ethical frameworks

Duty based (or 'deontology')

This examines the motives and intentions of the action. Each individual has duties and obligations to others. Any rights possessed occur as a result of that duty. Conscience and motive of the person carrying out those actions are important.

Rights based

People inherently have 'rights' and duties occur in order to maintain these rights. However, true rights can only be held by those capable of making autonomous decisions.

Goals based (or 'utilitarian')

The action itself is viewed from the perspective of its outcome. The ultimate purpose of morality is to increase the sum of pleasure/happiness. Therefore, the action is good if the outcome is good and vice versa. Often found attractive to the medical profession as harm/benefit calculations for the individual patient are often made in clinical practice.

Other terms or 'four principles' often used in ethical discussion

1 **Beneficence:** Using medical skills to do good, e.g. GMC injunction to 'put your patient's interests first'

2 **Non-maleficence:** From the Hippocratic tradition of 'first of all, do no harm'

3 **Respect for autonomy:** Autonomy means 'self-rule'. There is a basic human right to bodily integrity that underpins consent. Doctors promise to respect confidentiality

4 **Justice:** To do with fairness, payment systems, universal access to the NHS and rationing

---

Figure 19.1 shows a diagrammatic representation of the relationship between medicine, law and ethics with a dilemma about how to act in the centre. 'Is x possible?' is a clinical question, whether the signing of a sick note, the prescribing of a medication, a minimally invasive procedure or major operation. The clinical facts and research literature are all important in working out the benefits and harms of the action.

It is an entirely separate question to ask 'Is x legal?' For example, infertility activities are regulated by the Human Fertilisation and Embryology Authority. Inserting a large number of embryos might increase the chance of pregnancy, but can be illegal (depending on the age of the recipient). Prescribing penicillin to a penicillin allergic patient may lead to a civil claim in negligence due to falling below a legal standard of care. Lastly, just because an action might be technically possible and legal, does not make it right (or, at least, good enough).

In gynaecological practice, it is rare to have a day without coming across a challenging clinical situation that tests these boundaries (Box 19.4). We often react to situations before we have time to reflect about the ethics involved. Sometimes it is only afterwards that the gravity and sensitivity of a situation is realized. This emphasizes the need for reflective practice; to hone the intuitive skills, relevant medical knowledge and character development.

Ethics and law are intertwined. Medical ethics is about the highest achievable standard of behaviour, whereas law deals with the lowest acceptable practice. Law is invoked to limit personal and professional judgements and freedoms when personal and professional ethics are not enough. Professional codes

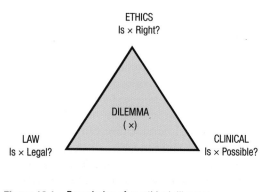

Figure 19.1   Boundaries of an ethical dilemma.

- Genital surgery on infants to 'correct' intersex conditions
- Underage sex and contraceptive advice
- Adolescent confidentiality
- Partner notification about sexually transmitted infection
- Abortion
- Antenatal screening
- Termination for congenital anomalies
- Screening for viral infections in pregnancy
- Pre-implantation diagnosis
- Fertility treatment at increasing age
- Multiple embryo transfer
- Assisted conception for same sex couples
- Female genital mutilation
- Cosmetic 'request' surgery

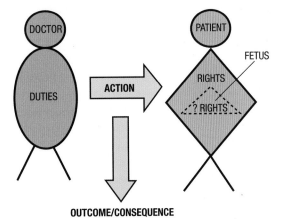

Figure 19.2 Doctor–patient relationship: the interaction between duty, rights and consequences.

One dilemma in detail: abortion

Legality of abortion

If a man kicks a woman in the abdomen to try and end the pregnancy, that is a serious crime. Abortion is illegal under the 1861 Offences against the Person Act, excepting if certain circumstances pertain that make it legal. Procuring a miscarriage is an intentional crime which could result in a mandatory life sentence for the woman and doctor. The 1967 Abortion Act placed the responsibility for determining the legality of abortion with doctors. There is no legal right to 'abortion on demand'. Two registered practitioners must be of the opinion made in good faith that one of the clauses (Table 19.1) has been fulfilled, and the abortion must be performed on licensed premises and notified.

Ethical issues in abortion

The central ethical question in abortion is the moral worth of the fetus: Does the fetus have full, some or no moral status? Even if it has full moral status, equivalent to the mother, when would the rights of the mother override those of the fetus (e.g. the right to kill in self-defence if the pregnancy threatens her life)?

The moral arguments are simple only for those people holding the extreme (and consistent) views that:

- Abortion is *always* morally wrong: because life starts at conception and no human being has the right to take life (even in the case of rape or self-defence). Abortion is equivalent to murder.

of conduct act as a bridge between the ethical and legal dimensions encouraging consistency between practitioners, allowing for public accountability and transparency.

Analysing ethical dilemmas

When looking at any doctor–patient interaction, there are two significant moral players: the doctor and the patient. There may be other third parties of moral significance, particularly the fetus in pregnancy. Each has their own moral value and a relationship exists between them (Figure 19.2).

There are the duties of the doctor and the rights of the patient(s). Then there is the maximizing of the good outcome for the patient from any situation. Sometimes it may be impossible to find a decision where all these three tenets are met.

When making challenging decisions it may be useful to consider the legal and ethical dimensions. It is prudent to be informed about relevant professional guidelines. This builds on reflective practice and creates a personal dialogue. It helps a doctor mount a reasoned argument as to why a particular course of action is followed. If a balanced argument is presented and the actions were within the law, doctors can feel more secure about their decisions. Often, a person's actual actions and opinions may lie in the middle of the three boundaries in Figure 19.1.

Table 19.1 Clauses of the Abortion Act 1967 (modified by Human Fertilisation and Embryology Act 1994)

A	The continuance of the pregnancy would involve risk to the life of the pregnant woman greater than if the pregnancy was terminated
B	The termination is necessary to prevent grave permanent injury to the physical and mental health of the pregnant woman
C	The continuance of the pregnancy would involve risk, greater than if the pregnancy were terminated, of injury to the physical or mental health of the pregnant woman
D	The continuance of the pregnancy would involve risk, greater than if the pregnancy were terminated, of injury to the physical or mental health of any existing children of the family of the pregnant woman
E	There is substantial risk that if the child were born it would suffer from physical or mental abnormalities as to be seriously handicapped

A woman has a duty to her innocent and vulnerable fetus which will grow into a child that has interests that need protecting regardless of her preferences or well-being.

- Abortion is *never* morally wrong: No woman should be forced to use her body against her will. At no time before birth is the fetus an independent human being. The functions of personhood are what gives a human being full moral status. Therefore the fetus does not have any 'right to life', and does not require the same absolute respect for life as the mother.

It is not possible for these two views to be reconciled. Many disrespectful and heated arguments take place without addressing the central issues of moral worth, women's rights and how to handle these disagreements within any society.

Some believe that anything less than 'abortion on demand' is an attack on women's rights to self-determination. They trust that women will make good decisions if allowed and find time limits and clauses too restrictive. It is known that women terminate less frequently with increasing gestation (e.g. for the same congenital anomaly diagnosed in the first or second trimester). Women can present late due to adverse social circumstances and they may have to continue the pregnancy. It is important for doctors to discuss fostering and adoption, although they are difficult options for all parties.

Since 1967, there have been regular attempts to change the law and there are continuing peaceful efforts to reduce time limits and indications. In the United States especially, there have been some more extreme and even violent attempts to stop abortion; e.g. picketing of women attending clinics and the shooting of doctors performing abortions.

Abortion was illegal not so long ago in the UK, and remains so in many countries in the world. Even if illegal, unsafe abortions still take place, and contribute significantly to the maternal death rate. Maternal mortality has been shown to rise and fall directly with changes in abortion law in many countries. Gynaecologists have usually been in the forefront of contraception provision and abortion liberalization as they deal with the complications of unsafe abortion and rate women's lives highly.

Most people do not hold extreme views, but believe the fetus has some moral status (but not as much as mothers) that increases with gestation. The arguments then range about what abortions are acceptable before certain time limits. When is it that the fetus begins to have moral worth? Does the acquisition of worth and rights occur suddenly – i.e. from none to full at some point such as conception, implantation, quickening (first noticing of movements), viability or birth? Or does the worth of fetuses increase gradually, or stepwise, with biological development? Then, some abortion decisions made at 10 weeks of gestation may be acceptable but would be unacceptable at 20 weeks or beyond the threshold of viability at 24 weeks.

With such divergent and controversial views, how can abortion law be framed justly? In the UK, Parliament leaves abortion decisions to the private discussions between medical professionals and women, relying on professional good sense.

These private discussions take place within a public framework of oversight and the threat of criminal punishment if the lines are overstepped. Individuals have personal views on abortion but have a duty of care to provide information and advice as honestly and impartially as possible. As long as the legal parameters above are fulfilled and the woman has made an autonomous informed decision, no criticism will be attached to the doctor, despite the particular ethical dilemmas.

The duty of the doctor is to provide safe and impartial care to the woman within the law. Out of respect for deeply held and religious views, abortion is the only procedure in medicine to which doctors can have a formal conscientious objection. Patients do not know the political or religious views of their doctors, and to impose one's own personal views on a patient would be a misuse of the trusting doctor–patient relationship. Thus, if a woman requests a termination, she must be referred to someone who can discuss and explain all the options. No doctor is forced to engage in abortion. However, there is still a responsibility to care for the woman if any complications should arise from the procedure.

In a pluralistic society, such as the UK, with law that both protects fetuses and permits abortion, the moral approach can be seen as lying between the extremes, with a gradualist approach to fetal moral worth.

Conclusion

The psychosocial and ethical challenges in gynaecology are complex. Developing the skills to sensitively explore deeper problems in women's lives enables the building of a more trusting relationship. This involves self-reflection about one's own attitudes and consultation style. Every woman's story is different and worth disentangling. This may reveal the cause of, or reaction to, her symptoms. It may seem daunting initially but awareness of the issues involved and a sympathetic approach are the first steps to giving the best medical care in the context of that individual.

COMMON GYNAECOLOGICAL PROCEDURES

Hysteroscopy

Hysteroscopy involves passing a small-diameter telescope, either flexible or rigid, through the cervix to directly inspect the uterine cavity. Excellent images can be obtained. A flexible hysteroscope may be used in the outpatient setting, with carbon dioxide as a filling medium. Rigid instruments employ circulating fluids and therefore can be used to visualize the uterine cavity even if the woman is bleeding.

Indications

Any abnormal bleeding from the uterus can be investigated by hysteroscopy, including:

- postmenopausal bleeding,
- irregular menstruation, intermenstrual bleeding and postcoital bleeding,
- persistent menorrhagia,
- persistent discharge,
- suspected uterine malformations,
- suspected Asherman's syndrome.

Complications

- Perforation of the uterus.
- Cervical damage – if cervical dilatation is necessary.
- If there is infection present, hysteroscopy can cause ascent.

An operating hysteroscope can also be used to resect endometrial pathology such as fibroids and polyps.

Laparoscopy

Laparoscopy allows visualization of the peritoneal cavity. This involves insertion of a needle called a

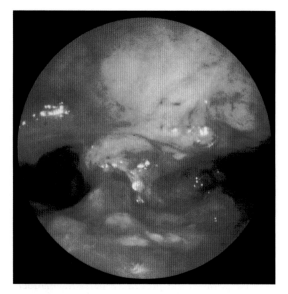

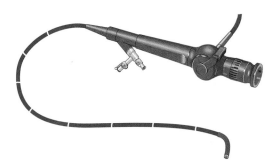

Figure 1   Flexible fibreoptic hysteroscope.

Figure 2   Hysteroscopic view of endometrial cavity.

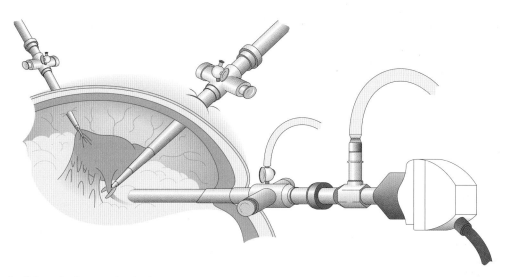

Figure 3   Schematic diagram showing laparoscope.

Veress needle into a suitable puncture point in the umbilicus. This allows insufflation of the peritoneal cavity with carbon dioxide so that a larger instrument can be inserted. The majority of instruments used for diagnostic laparoscopy are 5mm in diameter, and 10mm instruments are used for operative laparoscopy. More recently, a 2mm laparoscope has become available.

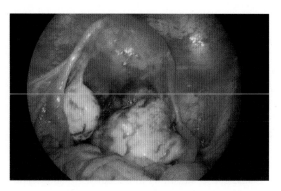

Figure 4   Laparoscopic view of bilateral endometriomas.

Indications

- Suspected ectopic pregnancy.
- Undiagnosed pelvic pain.
- Tubal patency testing.
- Sterilization.

Operative laparoscopy can be used to perform ovarian cystectomy or oophorectomy and to treat endometriosis with cautery or laser. Reversal of sterilization is also possible using laparoscopy.

Complications

Complications are uncommon, but include damage to any of the intra-abdominal structures, such as bowel and major blood vessels. The bladder is always emptied prior to the procedure to avoid bladder injury. Incisional hernia has been reported.

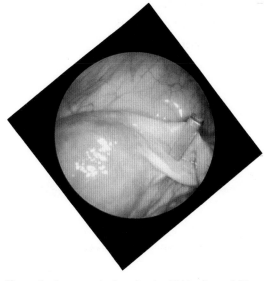

Figure 5   Laproscopic view showing Fishie clip on right Fallopian tube.

Abdominal and vaginal hysterectomy

Vaginal hysterectomy is associated with a much quicker recovery than abdominal hysterectomy and is preferred for that reason. However, vaginal hysterectomy is not indicated when there is malignancy, as the ovaries often need to be removed and lymph nodes examined and sampled. If the uterus is larger than that of a 12-week pregnancy and has outgrown the pelvis, an abdominal hysterectomy is usually preferred and is thought to be safer. The main reason vaginal hysterectomy is associated with faster recovery is the lack of abdominal incision.

Most abdominal hysterectomies are performed through a Pfannenstiel incision, which is a low (bikini line) suprapubic transverse incision. Patients recover more quickly from this incision than from than a midline incision and the cosmetic result is more acceptable. For larger masses and malignancies, a midline incision is utilized.

Although a complete description of abdominal hysterectomy is outside the scope of this chapter, the procedure involves taking three pedicles:

- the infundibulopelvic ligament, which contains the ovarian vessels,
- the uterine artery,
- the angles of the vault of the vagina, which contain vessels ascending from the vagina; the ligaments to support the uterus can be taken with this pedicle or separately.

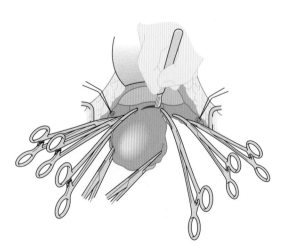

Figure 6   Total abdominal hysterectomy with clamps on.

In the vaginal hysterectomy, the same steps are taken but in the reverse order.

Indications for abdominal hysterectomy

- Uterine, ovarian, cervical and Fallopian tube carcinoma.
- Pelvic pain from chronic endometriosis or chronic pelvic inflammatory disease where the pelvis is frozen and vaginal hysterectomy is impossible.
- Symptomatic fibroid uterus greater than 12-week size.

Indications for vaginal hysterectomy

- Menstrual disorders with a uterus less than 12 weeks in size.
- Microinvasive cervical carcinoma.
- Uterovaginal prolapse.

Complications

Specific complications of hysterectomy include:

- haemorrhage
- ureteric injury
- bladder and bowel injury.

Cystoscopy

Cystoscopy involves passing a small-diameter telescope, either flexible or rigid, through the urethra into the bladder. Excellent images of both these structures can be obtained. A cystoscope with an operative channel can be used to biopsy any abnormality, perform bladder neck injection, retrieve stones and resect bladder tumours.

Indications

- Haematuria.
- Recurrent urinary tract infection.
- Sterile pyuria.
- Short history of irritative symptoms.

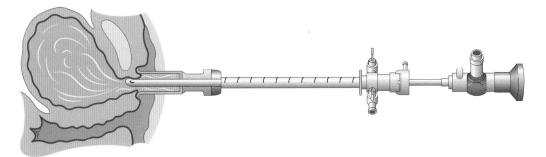

Figure 7   Diagram showing the cystoscopic procedure.

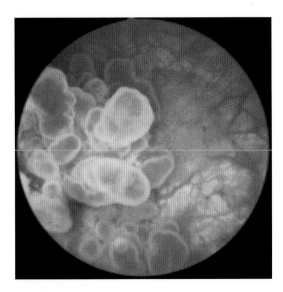

Figure 8   Cystoscopic view of bladder papilloma.

- Suspected bladder abnormality (e.g. diverticulum, stones, fistula).
- Assessment of bladder neck.

Complications

- Urinary tract infection.
- Rarely, bladder perforation.

MEDICO-LEGAL ASPECTS OF GYNAECOLOGY

Litigation

Litigation has become a major feature of medical practice over the last two decades. Not only has the frequency of claims escalated, but also the basis for these claims has changed. Complications that were once viewed as acceptable hazards of common surgical procedures are now commonly the source of litigation. In other words, the Bolam Principle that has provided the guidelines for judgements about negligence in the past is no longer being applied. The fact that actions taken by a doctor may be considered to be reasonable by a significant number of medical colleagues is no longer always a defence, and in reality a complication is increasingly taken as evidence that there has been substandard practice. It is therefore important, both as a basis for good practice and to avoid litigation, to minimize the risk of complications.

Case records are medico-legal documents and whilst they are of great importance in the general care of the patient, they also provide the basis for the defence of a case in medico-legal claims. Case records should be kept for a minimum of 7 years in gynaecology and 25 years in obstetrics. It is essential to remember that case records may be scrutinized in a court case line by line, so they should contain nothing that is not accurate, factual and contemporaneous.

All entries in case notes must be dated and signed in a legible fashion. Too often it is impossible to decipher the signature after a case note entry and, as medical staff in the training grades commonly move on to other jobs, it can be subsequently very difficult to trace the personnel in an individual case. The same principle applies to entries that are made into computer records, although it may be easier to trace the authors through their access codes.

If it is necessary to alter or modify an entry in the case notes, it is important to countersign and date any modifications so that the alteration is seen to be a deliberate act. Important reports, such as histopathology reports, should be signed and dated at the time of receipt and when they are placed in the records to demonstrate that the report has been noted and the appropriate action taken.

Consent

The following is the legal definition of consent as laid down by the Medical Defence Union.

The competent adult patient has a fundamental right to give, or withhold, consent to examination, investigation or treatment. This right is founded on the moral principle of respect for autonomy.

An autonomous person has the right to decide what may or may not be done to him (or her). Any treatment or investigation or, indeed, even deliberate touching, carried out without consent may amount to battery. This could result in an action for damages, or even criminal proceedings, and in a finding of serious professional misconduct by the healthcare professional's registration body.

Consent must be informed or it becomes invalid. In obtaining consent, it is important that the patient understands the nature of any procedure that is to be performed and the attendant risks of that procedure.

In most instances, consent is obtained in writing, but consent may be implied by the patient's actions or by oral consent. Material risks must be made clear to the patient and the consent form must be signed before premedication is given. However, there is no longer any certainty about what constitutes a 'material risk'.

The consent form should be signed by the patient and, ideally, by the surgeon who will perform the procedure. It must, however, be emphasized that consent forms are only of value if it is evident that the consent is informed.

Consent for minors

The legal age for consent for medical and surgical treatment is 16 years or above. Under the age of 16 years, the situation is more complex. When an under-age child consents to treatment, the doctor may proceed with that treatment. If the child refuses treatment, that refusal can be over-ridden by someone with parental authority.

INDEX

Note: Page numbers in **bold** refer to diagrams and information contained in tables and boxes.